I'm Peeing as Fast as I Can

A Support Group's True Stories of
Bladder Pain Syndrome/Interstitial Cystitis

A urologist, a nurse, and twenty Citrus Valley IC Support Group partners share more than a decade of combined experience dealing with Bladder Pain Syndrome/Interstitial Cystitis (BPS/IC).

Edward L. Davis, M.D. Diplomat American Board of Urology
Edited by: Josephine Davis, R.N., B.S.N., C.R.C.

Publisher's Note

The material contained in this publication is neither intended nor implied to be given as medical advice. This publication is not intended to serve as a substitute for medical care or consultation with your physician. The information contained herein has been gathered from multiple sources with the intention of sharing a wide-range of information. If you have additional questions, please consult your physician or medical practitioner.

Various trademarked products and names are printed in this book. They are used in an editorial fashion with no intention of infringement of the trademark.

Care has been taken to verify the accuracy of the information presented by each contributor; each describes their therapeutic practices and how it related to their medical care. The contributors, editors, and publisher, however, are not responsible for errors or oversight or any consequences from application of the information in this book, and make no guarantee, express or implied, with respect to the contents of this publication.

Each individual insight into Bladder Pain Syndrome/Interstitial Cystitis (BPS/IC) may have a contributor presenting his or her drug related treatment and at times drug dosage. As with all medical intervention associated with medication and devices, the physician, pharmacist, package insert, and common sense guides the patient. We urge the reader for their safety to discuss any of the medical treatment choices addressed by the contributors to this book be a discussion with their physician(s).

The following are personal insights into the search for a treatment for BPS/IC that would bring about some measure of success. Ongoing research, government regulations, discovery of drug reactions information is ever evolving. It is the responsibility of the health care provider to determine the Food and Drug Administration (FDA) recommended use and/or precautions.

About the Authors

Edward Davis, M.D.

Edward Davis, M.D. graduated from the University of Missouri and completed his internship and urology residency at Los Angeles County/University of Southern California Medical Center. He has practiced his urology specialty in Glendora, California since graduation, and received his board certification by the American Board of Urology more than 35 years ago.

Dr. Davis with his wife, Josephine, formed the Citrus Valley Interstitial Cystitis Support Group in 2000. The focus of the group is education and problem solving as it relates to Painful Bladder Syndrome (PBS) historically known as IC.

Dr. Davis's interest in Painful Bladder Syndrome was the foundation for the start of Citrus Valley Medical Research. The majority of the studies have as a goal the control of BPS/IC symptoms that often focuses on the pelvic pain that is not easily controlled.

Dr. Davis's experience in urology and as a Colonel in the United States Air Force and California Air Guard, retired, helped him understand the need for a plan to direct action toward a set goal; this means with planning there is the best chance for the realization of the success. BPS/IC frustrating features can take charge of life; BPS/IC demands an individual work on the return of control prepared with the knowledge and support.

The Citrus Valley IC Support Group uses the words "Challenge, Partnership, Commitment" to describe the key elements to help bring calm out of chaos. Dr. Davis credits a person's understanding of the challenge, knowing the need for support, and making the commitment to follow the first step with a second as the building blocks of progress. These specific words of direction are the basis of this book along with shared personal accounts and shared wisdom.

Josephine Davis, R.N., B.S.N., C.R.C.

Josephine Davis, BS RN graduated from Shadyside Hospital School of Nursing, Pittsburgh, Pennsylvania, Pasadena City College, Pasadena, California and she earned her B.S.N, from University of St Francis, Los Angeles program. Her Southern California nursing career began at the University of Southern California, Los Angeles Medical Center. Mrs. Davis works at Citrus Valley Urologic Medical Group in the BPS/IC Clinic with two patient advocates. Jo has more than 14 years of interaction with men and women with BPS/IC. She has learned as much as she has taught from each patient and member of the support group about the impact BPS/IC has on life.

Jo and Ed Davis have been married for forty-five years. They have two sons, two daughters-in-law, and two grandchildren. Their home is in Glendora, California.

The title of the book, "I'm Peeing as Fast as I Can," is based on the interchange between two women separated by a public restroom stall door. Jo is on the work side of the door struggling to complete voiding and finding that her bladder is again not cooperating in her efforts. The symptoms of urinary urgency, frequency, and pelvic pain produce reaction mix of frustration, helplessness, and anger and are the emotional description of BPS/IC.

This chance restroom meeting was the day Jo decided she needed to meet her bladder challenge and have a plan of action. Jo's personal story grew into the series of support group stories. What originated as a self-discovery commitment has become an education and a path of learning to share about BPS/IC.

Contents

Forwards Worth Reading

Support Group's Discovery & Recovery Experiences

Where Do I Go From Here?

Acknowledgements

A Physician's View of BPS/IC – What I think
Edward L. Davis, M.D.

When I graduated from the University of Missouri Medical School, I thought I knew everything. With each passing year of medical practice, I am humbled by how much I need to learn. I have been acutely aware of the difficulty that physicians have in making a change in medical care even when the frustration of failure to help our patients keeps hitting us in the face; Bladder Pain Syndrome/Interstitial Cystitis fits that description of hitting multiple medical roadblocks with unfortunate precision.

For many years, men and women came to my office seeking help for urinary urgency, frequency, and pelvic pain. My treatment and support was based on standard "good" medical practice, but I knew they needed more. Professional medical knowledge was limited about Interstitial Cystitis. IC rated a short paragraph in the medical textbooks. IC was relegated to a profile of affecting mainly, elderly, neurotic women and men who had a mysterious bacterial cause for testicular and prostate pain. Both sexes were sadly dismissed.

My frustration increased over the years because the little scientific information available about IC was seeped in antiquated literature and myths. My medical colleagues were just as oblivious as to the multiple combinations of the symptoms of IC. I recognized how patients were bounced from one medical specialist to another without receiving any help. I was part of that chain of doctor visits.

I saw a glimmer of forward thinking from the pharmaceutical company, Alza in 1997. Alza was the first to address IC as a distressing and life altering disorder; and yes, they did have a medication to sell, pentosan polysulfate sodium or Elmiron made from beech tree bark. Elmiron as an oral medication had the unique ability to coat the bladder lining and Federal Drug Administration (FDA) trials had proven it safe and effective to quiet IC distressing bladder symptoms.

As we move toward another generation of time passing, what Alza discovered as resistance to their Elmiron, marketing campaign remains true about Interstitial Cystitis, specifically: (a) IC continues to be a relatively poorly understood disease process and has a low awareness of recognition; therefore affective treatment remains a matter of luck. (b) A reluctance of many physicians to treat IC that proves the pharmaceutical industries substantial attempts to address this phenomena of the IC blind spot through medical education have been a tepid success.

This lack of interest of medicine in pelvic pain of bladder origin is a combination of four formidable forces:

(1) *There is no definitive test for BPS/IC.* Research and development at the university level or from the National Institute of Health (NIH) or the pharmaceutical industry have not produced a means of testing. There have been promising directions such as urine showing a unique antiproliferative factor (APF) and another with a protein marker, but either the complicated nature of testing or the inconsistent validity of the results compounded by the lack of funding has stopped any progress.

(2) *The general low level of knowledge and awareness about IC in our general population.* When did you ever see or hear anyone having an open discussion about BPS/IC on commercial or cable radio or television? We may wonder about the legitimate nature of many of the media's causes, but as direct advertising has proven, getting the word out is necessary to beginning a spirited dialogue that filters to both the general public and physicians.

(3) *The surgical specialties of urology and gynecology, the key word being "surgery" are designated as the point guards for bladder problems.* I was reminded that I had stated with great emphasis that all diseased parts should be in a specimen bottle to be cured; in short I was saying that as a surgeon my best effort is given to a focused procedure and then moving on to the next surgical need.

(4) *BPS/IC is a chronic condition that requires time to manage.* BPS/IC is a medical problem that has, because of anatomical location and history, been required to be diagnosed and treated by surgical specialties.

(5) *What I see on the inside.*

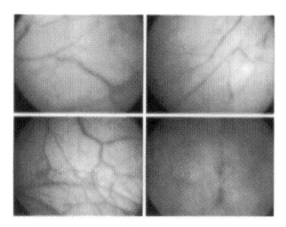

The above images show what a normal bladder membrane looks like.

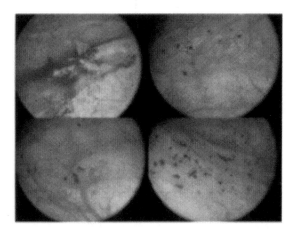

The above images show examples of a BPS/IC ulcerated bladder membrane.

Breakthroughs

There have been random breakthroughs such as the advertising executive who thought up *over active bladder (OAB)*. This advertising label gave millions of men and women a reason for why their lives are impacted by frequent voiding, lack of a good night sleep, and millions of doses of antibiotics for a bacteria that is never found in urine specimens sent to a lab for culture. Though OAB has been a side note of discussions about BPS/IC the symptoms and impact of OAB are often the stepping-stones to the level of bladder & pelvic pain that is diagnosed as BPS/IC.

One giant step in BPS/IC care that has happened over the past five years is the medical and pharmaceutical recognition that having the bladder lining repaired is often only half the healing process. As the millions of nerve endings in the damaged bladder wall are assaulted by often multiple years caustic exposure the nerves remain in an overactive state and continue to cause flares even a person has made the dietary and life changes to aide healing. Enter a new line of BPS/IC medications that began with seizure disorder medication, Neurontin; then refined to the product Lyrica. Yet once again these are medication tools that have their side effects.

It is well known in the patient community that often migraine headaches, fibromyalgia, irritable bowel, and BPS/IC can come in sets or an entire package of misery to one person. Also well known, because it is experienced first-hand, is the sensitivity or what is commonly labeled allergic response that occurs seasonally, under dietary or environmental circumstances that can set off the chain of events that is called a painful bladder/pelvic flare. The nerve pain component of BPS/IC is huge; research is just beginning to understand about this facet of symptom control without the use of narcotics.

Am I smarter about how to care for a BPS/IC patient? Yes. I can tell you that in the past fourteen years there have been true strides in our practice about taking control of BPS/IC, solving each individual's IC mystery, advising how to take charge and to begin recovery. We have a BPS/IC clinic that includes patient advocates with direct understanding of BPS/IC, as well as a research team to develop protocols and direct patients to research studies.

The following are insights into BPS/IC and the concluding "What I think" lists come from people who know that from denial can come self-discovery, from despair can come a sense of purpose, from frustration can come progress, and with common sense and perseverance can come recovery. This book is here to help support your recovery.

Edward L. Davis, M.D

A Nurse's View of Recovery – Lesson One
Jo Davis R.N., B.S.N., C.R.C.

Glendora, California is a small town; over the past fourteen years of Citrus Valley IC Support Group meetings, the contact list has never been less than three hundred names. I use to think Glendora must be ground zero for BPS/IC until I participated in the Rand Corporation's, Santa Monica, California, first statistical study titled the "Prevalence of Symptoms of Bladder Pain Syndrome/Interstitial Cystitis among Adult Females in the United States. (Published in J. Urol. 2011 August; 186(2): 540-544) The opening sentence comes right to the point, "Bladder pain syndrome/interstitial cystitis is a poorly understood condition that can cause serious disability." The Rand conclusion translated into 3.3 to 7.9 million United States women 18 years old or older with BPS/IC symptoms.

The Rand report pointed out that "symptoms and severity and impact were comparable to those adult women that had been diagnosed. But only 9.7% of the women reported being assigned a bladder pain syndrome/interstitial cystitis diagnosis." This means when we report to a physician the life altering BPS/IC symptoms, of urinary urgency, frequency, and pelvic pain, less than 10% of us has ever had a medical evaluation that identified bladder lining inflammation, thinning, and/or ulceration as the cause. These are powerful statistics because it indicates that without an accepted test for BPS/IC our medical evaluation falls in to the category of "diagnosis of exclusion" or if it's not anything else maybe it's BPS/IC.

An important point must be made now – BPS/IC does not begin with an evil spell cast on some females at the age of eighteen, it does not skip men or children. WebMD states that 55% of the U.S. population tests positive to one or more allergens. Allergens are part of the complex inflammatory response that damages the bladder lining; the BPS/IC bladder lining struggles to repair the protective coating so that the caustic effects of urine do not bring more BPS/IC symptoms and damage.

The search for answers to resolve the pelvic pain caused by our bladder lining erosion is the reason for publishing these revealing stories about Bladder Pain Syndrome/Interstitial Cystitis (BPS/IC.) The aim is to help make sense of why we spend so much time in the toilet and so much of our lives fighting the storm of symptoms that have the initials of BPS/IC. Twenty members of Citrus Valley

Interstitial Cystitis Support Group, Glendora, responded to my request for their accounts of coming to terms with pelvic pain when a damaged bladder lining is diagnosed as the cause. They have written about the search to find their individual paths of resolution of BPS/IC symptoms and what they discovered during the journey.

By way of email exchanges, you will meet Jan, wife, mother, teacher, and runner; she went from knowing only the medical label for her pelvic pain to understanding how to take greater control of her symptoms. Our conversations are a diary that began with confusion and misery to regaining a sense of positive and realistic momentum.

My awareness for the need to share personal experiences dealing with BPS/IC from our Glendora based Citrus Valley Support Group began with my encounter with reality in the restroom of the Angeles baseball stadium. It was the seventh inning stretch; I'm hurrying to get to a stall before having to stand in line. Again, I find myself staring at the business side of scratched metal bathroom door with a latch that almost locks. This is my third visit. I think relax, the nagging pain will go away if I void just one more drop; I think "Lord why me?"

The door is pushed. A voice connected to a pair of blue tennis shoes says, "Are you done, there are a lot of us out here waiting. What is your problem? Are you alright? I really have to go. This is not your private toilet."

The door handle moves, and I know it would take only a slight push to have MS "Blue Shoes" in my lap. This is when I sob, "I'm peeing as fast as I can."

There is a one, two beat of silence and the woman wearing the blue shoes replied, "I hear you sister. I know what you mean. Take a deep breath; sometimes it helps me to press on my stomach. You will be O.K. Sorry, I really have to go."

In that stadium restroom exchange was the exasperated thoughts I lived with; then came understanding and support from an anonymous but understanding voice through a closed door.

I have worked with the Citrus Valley Urologic Medical Group, BPS/IC Clinic and Support Group for a long time. I am grateful to be able to listen and learn from people like those who wrote the following accounts and share with you the revelation that there are many of us with BPS/IC and peeing as fast as we can.

Jo Davis, R.N, B.S.N., C.R.C.

Support Group's Discovery & Recovery Experiences

1. A Nurse's View of Recovery: What I Have Learned Lesson Two

I am Jo Davis, wife, mom, and grandmother. The initials after my name designate Registered Nurse with a Bachelor of Science degree and also a certification in clinical research. Since 2001, I have been employed by the Citrus Valley Urologic Medical Group and Citrus Valley Medical Research. My focus is the Support Group, the IC Clinic, and clinical research.

How the support group and this book began:

I backed into a lifestyle and career shift after attending a lunchtime in-service program. In January 2000, my husband, Ed Davis, M.D. invited me to a presentation for medical personal about a bladder condition called Interstitial Cystitis (IC). To this day, I do not know if it was by chance or that he planned to have me listen to a symptom list that matched mine. I would ask or demand my antibiotics and clutched a heating pad to my lower abdomen, and rolled over in pelvic pain more times than I can remember.

Ed would ask me to have a specimen of my urine sent to the laboratory for culture to check if I really had a bladder infection; I would step over that request. My answers were a mix of: (1) I am a nurse (the sweeter version of "back off"); (2) I've handled this monthly increased need to void and vague pelvic pain with antibiotics for years. And my fall back position, (3) I know I have a "nervous and small" bladder because my mother told me it runs in the family. Live with it. Family wisdom was to have an aisle seat and always know the closest location to the bathroom. How can you argue with this logic?

The hospital in-service talk had a slide presentation that showed a bladder in flames. It took my breath away and in a reflex action I clutched my belly. I noticed that around the room there were nods of recognition. When the discussion turned to multiple courses of antibiotics for urinary tract infection symptoms and the repeated use of pain medication with only a chance of temporary pain relief, I knew I was about to be educated about what was going on in my body.

Ed realized that there were both men and women coming to his office seeking help for urinary urgency, frequency, and pelvic pain. The treatment or support was based on standard "good" medical practice, but he knew they needed more. Medical knowledge was limited to the fact that the professional medical understanding about IC was a short paragraph in the textbooks. IC was relegated to mainly elderly, neurotic women, and sadly dismissed.

His frustration increased because there was so little information available about IC. His medical colleagues were as oblivious to IC and pelvic pain as he had been. Ed recognized how patients were bounced from one medical specialist to another without receiving help.

After the IC talk, Ed asked me to help him, one time and one time only, to start an IC support group. We began to meet in the very same room as the IC hospital presentation the following month, February 2000. Since then information about IC continues to improve. The number of valid treatment options is longer, yet the debate about the very existence of IC continues.

My involvement and learning has grown from support group volunteer and organizer to include employment at the urology and research medical offices. I say that Ed hired me because I know the *real* need to pee. This understanding has made it easier for me to appreciate the life changes that occur when defective systems take over our daily lives.

This is the book that started with a onetime only support meeting. It has expanded to this guide of information because the Citrus Valley IC Support Group was established as a place to learn. Our meetings feature medical specialists, nutritionists, and physical therapists as well as addressing psychological issues. The goal is to share experiences and common sense strategies to bring greater order into our lives.

The shared dilemmas, insights, solutions, advocacy, and partnerships of support are all in the list of meaningful words that add up to moving beyond just making it to the next day.

Our Support Group knows, on a person-by-person basis, that clitoral, vulvar, urethral, and prostate pain is often in the mix of IC symptoms. We often have bladder pain that makes itself known and is reflected in other parts of pelvic area and because of how the nerve supply runs from the lower back, thighs and even great toes.

A common question asked is "have we over reached by connecting all these conditions under bladder and/or pelvic pain? We do not think we have over reached because each of the symptoms of pelvic and pelvic floor is evident as nerve fibers become intensely activated. This book is a tool to understand how chronic pelvic pain and our bladders interact with pain fibers and techniques to bring balance back into our lives.

We recognize the impact of bladder, vulvar, urethral, clitoral, and prostate pain that ranges from the annoyance of urinary urge, frequency, and irritation to intense and often constant misery.

This BPS/IC, OAB, CP/COOS, VP and urethritis guide focuses on the information to make sense out of the alphabet soup of bladder, pelvic floor, and prostate conditions that have put us in a survival position.

Our support meetings have explored the many facets of bladder lining dysfunction from the anatomy, biology, medical, and patient/personal perspectives. As a support group we have become educated to the connections of Irritable Bowel Syndrome, Fibromyalgia, migraine, food, and environmental sensitivities that often intertwine with our pelvic pain.

Our support group is realistic. We know that one-size solutions do not fit all. What we have done is have our partnership of patients, physician, nurse, and patient advocates share with you what we have learned through trial, error, success, and listening.

The point of this book is to go beyond survival to recovery.

Jo Davis, R.N., B.S.N., C.R.C.

2. Bethany, age 28
What is BPS/IC? A Daughter Shares Her Discoveries

Background

Our recovery guide begins with a clear explanation of IC written by Bethany, She and her mother, Carol, have a partnership of support that is first a mother and daughter bond. Bethany understands IC from a family perspective. Carol has for many years been in the process of getting her life back from effects of BPS/IC. Bethany has been by her mom's side for painful flares, medical office appointments, emergency rooms visits when her mother's inability to urinate had risen to crisis levels, support group meetings, and the celebration of large and small successes that result from the pursuit of resolutions to pelvic pain.

The following is Bethany's exploration of IC and the information she shared on our Support Group's site that shows the depth of her involvement and learning about Interstitial Cystitis. As stated on the website, "Bethany has a personal understanding and knowledge of how IC spins your world."

Bethany Speaks, "What's in a Name?"
Bladder Pain Syndrome/Interstitial Cystitis (BPS/IC)

From the turn of nineteenth century the medical description of Interstitial Cystitis (IC): The lining of the bladder or "interstitium" and (2) being inflamed "cystitis" in short an inflamed bladder lining.

The historical view that IC is only a bladder problem boxed in 'medical profession thinking' for one hundred years. The growing body of scientific thought today is that interstitial cystitis is a set of pelvic symptoms shouting out that nerves have been recruited to bring about intense urinary urge, frequency, and pelvic pain.

IC describes the lining of the bladder but not the pain cycle. With the addition of the descriptive phrase "Bladder Pain Syndrome" (BPS), there is recognition of symptom patterns that need to be addressed. A syndrome means there is a set of signs that are present when pain has the bladder as the source.

Interstitial Cystitis is a chronic pelvic pain disease that directly involves and affects the bladder with an inflammatory process. Interstitial Cystitis is referred to as IC for short and often spoken of as pelvic pain caused by the bladder; throughout this paper both terms will be used.

The following is my understanding of IC. Common symptoms of Interstitial Cystitis include urinary frequency, urgency, and pelvic pain:

- Frequency is defined as having the urge to urinate many times during the day, and the cause of interrupted sleep during the night.

- Urgency is the immediate need to urinate. In IC, the protective bladder lining is thin and/or ulcerated; there can be constant pain from the acidic salts of urine touching these areas. If a person cannot go to the bathroom right away, urgency often causes pelvic pain as the bladder muscles go into spasm. These spasms can be so intense that it becomes impossible to void and catheterization (when a tube is put into the bladder to drain urine) is the only solution to bring relief. Until my mother learned to do her own catheterizations these painful episodes of urine retention were the reasons for many of our emergency room visits.

- The nerves located in the bladder cause IC pelvic pain. Although the bladder is about the size of your closed fist when not filled, it has an intense concentration of nerve fibers, and can cause severe and distressful pain throughout the entire body. When the bladder causes pain in other regions of the body, it is labeled "referred pain." Many IC patients experience referred pain up and down the lower back, kidney region, and down their legs, especially the right leg and right knee. Pain for IC patients typically centralizes itself in the lower abdomen, urethral, and vaginal areas.

Interstitial Cystitis overlaps several other diseases with its symptom patterns. These syndromes include Irritable Bowel Syndrome (IBS), vulvar vestibulitis known as vulvodynia, fibromyalgia, and migraine headaches. All of these diseases include in their description the words irritation, and inflammation that leads to nerve involvement and pain. To complicate matters, BPS/IC is not widely recognized or treated by the medical community; physicians continue to have limited knowledge of treatment plans to help a patient with IC.

Another red flag is that BPS/IC may be the cause of distress and pain during and/or after the sexual experience. The level of pelvic pain can and often does fluctuate with the menstrual cycle. For women, pelvic pain is usually associated with the reproductive organs and the reason why the gynecologist is often the first specialist to hear of lower abdominal agony and pelvic pain.

The list of miseries that are the banner of pelvic pain hit all the points that are described in medical literature when activated pain fibers produce painful urination, increase frequency, stimulate urgency, and discomfort on any level when going to the bathroom or between trips to the bathroom. If any of these symptoms are causing concern about your health, this is when a urology appointment should be made to evaluate the reason for your pelvic pain no matter what level of discomfort you have.

A urology evaluation begins with a urine culture to check for any infection and blood in the urine that may be the cause or part of the cause of IC like symptoms. This is urine specimen collected as a "clean catch" meaning the perianal area is wiped with special cleansing pads in one direction, with a change of pads for each wiping action. The urine stream is started and then stopped or urine is caught mid-stream to have some assurance that the specimen urine is not contaminated. At the laboratory level, the possibility of a bacterial infection will be documented and the correct antibiotic choices recommended.

A urology evaluation should begin with a urine culture to check for any infection that maybe the cause or part of the cause of IC symptoms. There is often a minute amount of blood in the urine that cannot be seen, but gives the signal that all is not well. This is where confusion often happens; a prescription for an antibiotic is written before knowing whether a bacterium is the cause of the inflammation leading to pelvic pain or the inflammatory response demonstrates the thinned bladder lining's struggle to regenerate cells which produce the vital protective covering of the bladder surface.

Urine directly from the bladder should be sterile, meaning no organisms. At the laboratory level the possibility of a bacterial infection will be confirmed or removed as a cause of the flare of IC symptoms. I know from my mother's experiences you can have both a urinary tract infection (UTI), commonly called a bladder infection that leads to a massive flare of IC symptoms. Also after the infection is resolved the flare symptoms may linger because the bladder lining is still inflamed.

A patient experiencing pain in the genital region can certainly be suffering from a number of other diseases that need to be eliminated as possibilities of causing IC symptoms such as bladder cancer has as a symptom of blood in the urine, tuberculosis, endometriosis, vaginal infections such as yeast, kidney involvement, and sexually transmitted diseases. This is why a specialist is needed to specifically define the cause of the urinary symptoms.

The cause of IC is not known. The inflammation that is noted when the bladder is examined appears to be bladder's response to urine. The needed replacement of the cells that make up the protective bladder's lining to push the urine away from the bladder wall is inadequate or missing, and the cycle of constant inflammation leads to exposed nerves in the bladder muscle and IC symptoms.

When it is determined that there is no bacterial infection, a cystoscopy, the procedure to insert a scope through the urethra to examine the bladder lining, is usually preformed. Additionally, a hydro distention is often part of the urologist or uro-gynecologist diagnostic process, meaning a large volume of water is used to increase the size of the bladder and this expands the surface for examination. Think of putting water into a balloon. This procedure should be done under anesthesia. I can tell you that my mother is a brave woman, but a cystoscopy with or without the hydrodistention would not be tolerated in an awake state.

The hydrodistention procedure that my mother had was under general anesthesia and allowed the urologist to look inside her bladder with a scope and camera to effectively make an assessment on the current condition of her bladder. This internal exam of the bladder helped in directing treatment and medication needs. Also I think the photos that were given to her showed us the inflammation in vivid color and were a visual explanation for her pelvic pain. A cystoscopy is also used to locate any ulcers, which cause bleeding and constant pain. Even with a direct view of the destruction or thinning of the bladder lining, the primary reason for the cause of IC is still a mystery.

Records show strong evidence of IC dating back to 1870 with written documentation from Lawson Tait's description of two cases of young women with bleeding bladder ulcers, pain on voiding, and urinary frequency. In 1914, Guy Hunner, M.D. discovered and named after him, "Hunner's Ulcer's" or ulcerations are open so wounds in the bladder lining. Hunner was an activist for surgical excision of the ulcers as the best treatment option for relief form pain. Hunner's Ulcers are the worst kind of bladder ulcerations that a patient can have, and the pain caused by these open sores is tremendous and often unbearable.

Any ulceration will cause pelvic pain, and blood loss ranges from minute to life threatening.

Despite IC being documented and treated since the late 19th century, there is no cure for IC. With all chronic health problems, each person must look for different coping methods and strategies. The fact is that everyone is different. The guide for moving forward toward recovery is recognizing your uniqueness.

The medical profession is beginning to realize that nerve involvement becomes activated when urine comes in contact with the muscle wall of the bladder; this can cause the flares that can stop daily life. The term "raw nerves" is true description of an IC flare.

Recovery Thoughts: Anyone who has worked on IC recovery knows that diet is watched closely, such as cutting down on eating acidic food, like tomatoes, pickles, spicy food, along with many other food items that cause a bad reaction in the bladder such as MSG (monosodium glutamate.) Another directive is the need to drink more water to dilute the urine so it is not so concentrated with salts that set off the unprotected nerve fibers.

Changes to diet, learning about rescues for both bladder pain and referred pain are key to gaining a sense of control. My mom has used ice/gel packs applied to her urethra and vaginal area (for safety always wrapped the gel ice pack so there won't be injury from the cold.) The cold helps reduce the inflammation that is at the center of a flare; it has been a great comfort and temporary pain reliever. Should you use heat? Yes, for the relief of pain that is referred to the back muscles and kidney area from the tension of bladder inflammation.

For stress reduction and reducing the acid environment in your body, use the time honored warm bath with baking soda added; about one cup and a soaking that will have the pelvic pain go down the drain. Your skin feels very smooth, and I think send a message from the brain to the muscles that it is O.K. to relax. You are letting your body take a big breath and the adrenaline flow as the pain eases. This is an observation of a daughter who has observed the tension build as pain become hours of agony. Two items that I have heard repeated over and over at doctor visits is the need to relax and have restful sleep; both suggestions are true but border on ludicrous when you are dealing with an IC flare. My mother says a warm baking soda bath does help.

Medications specifically for IC are limited. Elmiron (pentosan polysulfate sodium) for the past ten years has been the primary drug prescribed to bring Interstitial Cystitis under control. Almost all IC patients take Elmiron orally on a daily basis, and the use of Elmiron as a bladder instillation has been successful and tested in a clinical trial. My mom has had the Elmiron mixed with sterile normal saline and put directly in the bladder through a catheter; it is hypothesized to have Elmiron coat the bladder wall, creating a temporary bladder lining. This treatment helps protect the bladder wall nerves from acidic urine and other irritants that are in the bladder twenty-four hours a day. The thought is also that Elmiron directly instilled in the bladder puts a coating on directly on the bladder lining more rapidly than using oral alone.

Other drugs that have proved to provide relief include:

- Antidepressants, such as Zolfot; also prescribed is Elavil/amitriptyline though listed as an antidepressant it is used in low doses, as 10 mg and 25 mg for example, to control bladder spasms.
- For short term relief there is the analgesic Pyridium as a prescription or AZO over the counter medication; these two medications are an example of what is used when IC symptoms may be caused by infection and often used as a rescue for the times when inflammation causes bladder pain.
- Antihistamines help control the release of histamine chemicals and swelling by mast cells when they react to an environmental or food sensitivity or allergy; this release of histamine increases the level of pelvic pain by causing swelling and the activation of pain fiber. As an example of an often used antihistamine is the Allegra brand or the generic version fexofenadine. Allegra and Claritin (Loratadine) do not appear to cause drowsiness.
- Muscle relaxants are another category to help relieve pain.

Beyond oral medication, bladder instillations using DMSO (Dimethyl Sulfoxide) has a history of an FDA-approved treatment that brings for some patients brings temporary relief from pelvic pain. DMSO, medical grade, is instilled in the bladder with a catheter and held in the bladder for the length of time directed by the physician; then drained through a catheter. The hope is that the cycle of pain will be broken for a day or two and then not return to the same severe level of discomfort. Then there is the miracle of having a hydro distention and when the bladder is expanded with water the pain subsides for a prolong period for time

I know about many of the medications and treatment for IC because my mother was directly involved with all of them. The latest for my Mom was the Medtronic InterStim.

The InterStim has truly been a lifesaver for my mom. Because of the device, she does not have the severe retention problems; now her bladder gets the message that she needs to void more often, which causes her quite a bit of pain. Thankfully her doctors have found ways to help her cope with the burning pain and bladder spasms to keep it from getting out of control. Before the InterStim gave my Mom's bladder a giant sigh of relief, there was nothing like the pain and discomfort she had to experience from urinary retention and not being able to empty her bladder for hours on end. There is nothing in the world like the frustration of not being able to help your mother, who you love more than anything, stop the pain and find relief. I would feel so terrible when I had to take my Mom to the Emergency Room and they would drill her with questions and paperwork before finally getting her back into a room to drain her bladder and give her a much needed rescue treatment.

The only regret I can honestly think of regarding the InterStim implant is my Mom not getting it sooner. It was definitely a thoroughly thought-out, discussed and debated issue for at least a couple of years before deciding to give it the green light. A major factor for the delay was listening too much to outside opinions and reading too many horror stories. The sad thing about most medical devices or surgeries is that you can find thousands upon thousands of negative articles and reviews but it takes much more digging, research and time to uncover the positive feedback and success stories.

My advice to any patient that is considering getting an InterStim is to do your research, ask as many questions as you can possibly think of, and after that ask everything you forgot during the previous appointments. The more details and information you have, the more comfortable and confident you are going to be about having the InterStim surgery and living with a foreign device in your body.

When getting an InterStim implant, you will work closely with a Medtronic representative from the very first consultation to the follow-up appointments and after-care. The medical representatives we worked with throughout the InterStim process were attentive, responsive, willing to answer any and all questions, and always available when we needed them. They came to appointments when appropriate or were requested to be there and were present in the operating room during both the trial and permanent surgeries. The medical reps are responsible for making sure that the InterStim device works properly, is placed in the precise right location so that the patient receives the most relief possible and to answer any questions the surgeon may have concerning the device during the procedure. If a medical rep is needed at an appointment, even years after having the implant surgery, the doctor can contact them to be present to answer any questions or concerns the patient may have regarding their InterStim implant device.

When my Mom made the decision to definitely go ahead with getting an InterStim implant, it was a major disappointment and frustration to find out that her urologist was unable to perform the InterStim surgery because the insurance company and regulations currently in place do not allow urologists to do the procedure. For some unknown reason, only certain physicians are permitted to do the InterStim surgery and in our case, we had to find a qualified Pain Management Specialist. Fortunately, my Mom was already going to a rehabilitation institute for treatment of her severe migraines, back pain and chronic bladder pain. Since she first started going to Institute until now, she has been through approximately four doctors before the one she is currently seeing, became a permanent physician at the practice. He is personable, attentive and responsive, pays crucial attention to detail, takes his time, and truly cares about his patients. We never feel rushed during appointments, we feel comfortable approaching him with questions or concerns and we have always felt that he is an advocate for my Mom's health. On surgery/procedure days, he always comes in to talk to my mom and answer any questions she may have before she is wheeled into the operation room and has always checked in on her afterwards. He has fought the insurance company on her behalf, written letters when needed for work or travel needs and has been readily available when medications need to be refilled or adjusted. Dr. S. did a fantastic job with the InterStim. He was careful to monitor my Mom's comfort level and placement of the InterStim device so it would work properly and help her bladder release when she got the urge to pee.

It is extremely important when choosing a doctor to do your InterStim surgery that you feel completely comfortable with their overall manner and style of care, asking him or her any questions that may arise and feeling 100% confident about their ability to do the job well. Happy, confident and relaxed patients generally have both better results and recovery after the surgery is completed.

The InterStim surgery itself was relatively quick, uncomplicated and a lot simpler than my Mom had originally made it out to be. The anesthesiologist used enough sedation and anesthetic for my Mom to be relaxed and not aware of any pain, but light enough so that the doctor could ask my mom during the placement of the device if she could feel her bladder responding to the electronic stimulation. The surgery took a couple of hours and my Mom stayed in recovery for several more. We were at the hospital for the majority of the day and did not leave till very late in the evening. She was sore and in pain, but the surgery was definitely a success. During both times at a local hospital, the staff was outstanding and my Mom was made as comfortable as possible. My Mom and I like to refer to the hospital as the "Hilton". When we walked in for the first time, we were wondering where the concierge's desk was located!

After the InterStim implant trial surgery, the recovery period was short and not very painful. My Mom healed quite nicely and did not suffer from any post-operative complications. The recovery period after the permanent surgery, however; was a bit rough. My Mom was extremely sore and she experienced quite a bit of pain while healing. Her buttocks was very sore where the device was implanted along with the lumbar section of her back being very tender which is where the wires that communicate with the device are surgically inserted. As her patient advocate, I helped lift her up and down onto the bed, helped lower her down and up from the toilet, and did everything I could to help make her as comfortable as possible. I made sure she had ice, pain killer readily available and something to drink at all times to help her avoid getting cotton mouth from the anesthetic, painkillers and overall surgery aftermath. Every patient will react differently to the InterStim surgery, but having a patient advocate by your side to help with and do things for you that are suddenly a lot harder by yourself right after surgery is crucial to a successful recovery. It did not take long for the InterStim implant to prove its worth after the permanent surgery. In about 1-2 days, my Mom was going to the bathroom regularly throughout the day and her bladder was finally releasing the urine inside! She has praised Medtronic's InterStim implant ever since.

Something to keep in mind when considering the option of getting an InterStim implant is the upkeep it requires. The device has a battery life and must be charged when getting down about 50%. If the patient lets the battery die, surgery must be performed to replace or reset the device and this can cause unnecessary pain, discomfort, recovery time and possible complications. There is a charging device that must also be charged with a pack that plugs into an outlet. It is important to make sure this device stays at 100% as much as possible. This charger device is used to charge the implant inside the patient's body. In my Mom's case, her InterStim device is implanted in her right buttocks. She places the charging device on top of where the implant is located and adjusts it as needed so that it receives full charging strength. On the charging device's display screen, there are eight bars of "reception" as my Mom and I call it and the more bars you can get during charging, the faster the device will complete its charge. My Mom will either lie on the bed on her stomach or place the device on top of her buttocks, letting the InterStim charge while she rests or watches television. Another method is lying on her back on the bed against her pillows and placing the charging device against the InterStim implant, although this option makes it harder to keep the charging device against the InterStim. Charging her InterStim implant can become somewhat annoying; it can make the implant area get very warm, and my mom has frequently commented that it causes the area to hurt. After charging her InterStim device, my mom will often tell me she's very sore over the next couple of days from the charging session. Other then making sure everything stays charged and none of the battery levels run out, the upkeep for the InterStim device is actually pretty simple.

There is also a remote-like gadget that can turn your InterStim device on and off and controls how strong or weak you set the electronic stimulation coming from your InterStim. The Medtronic rep will initially program the InterStim with different settings and strength programs after your permanent surgery, depending on the severity of your condition and what you feel will help provide the most relief. This device takes regular AAA batteries and must be placed directly against the InterStim implant to change the unit's pulse setting. Another point to take into consideration when thinking about getting an InterStim is that when traveling, you must take all of this equipment with you for the charging, pulse control, turning the device on and off, etc. When going out every day on a regular basis to work, shopping, etc. all you need to take with you is the remote-like gadget that controls the electronic stimulation and allows you to turn off the device should it be necessary at any time.

Mark Twain said it best when he stated, "Against the assault of laughter, nothing can stand." Aside from the technical aspects, medical terminology, doctors, Medtronic reps, medications, surgeries and recovery periods, the one constant that has helped my Mother and me survive throughout this whole process has been keeping a sense of humor and a positive attitude. This may sound cliché to some, but without laughter and finding the silver lining in every situation, the entire process in getting my mom's InterStim implant from the very beginning involving discussions, weighing the good vs. the bad, consultations, insurance authorizations, appointments, anxiety, surgeries and after-care would have been overwhelming, beyond frustrating and downright depressing.

I refuse to let either myself or my Mother crawl into a hole and not continue enjoying life, no matter what uphill battle we might be enduring at the time. One of the easiest ways to keep this upbeat attitude and positive outlook is to constantly remind yourself that "It could be worse". You *could* be tied to a train track with a train barreling straight for you, but you're not. You *could* be stuck on the side of a mountain without food or water and no help for 200 miles in any direction, but you're not. And you *could* not have the care, guidance, help and support of doctors, family and friends, but you *do* have them. Remembering the positive things, big and small, and people you *do* have by your side is crucial to getting through the InterStim journey (and of course this applies to IC as well!).

Here are just a few amusing tidbits to hopefully bring a smile to your face and who knows, maybe even a laugh. A few years ago, I had managed to hide away enough money to surprise my mom with a trip to England. Well, this was probably the first big trip we had been on since my mom had her InterStim surgery and our first real test to traveling with her neurostimulator implant. She presented her medical device card to the officers at the security check and patiently waited to get the thorough pat down by the TSA. (When you have something like an InterStim, you cannot go through the normal security screeners due to the electromagnetic fields of the implant.) The funny part came on our way home when we departed London from Heathrow airport. She presented her medical device card and to make them understand what she had, she simply told them she had a pacemaker. When the security officer gave her the official pat down and came across the hard object in her right buttocks, my mom told her that what she was feeling was indeed her device. What the officer said next was priceless. She looked at my mom with a puzzled look and asked "Well how did it get way down here?" We still get a good laugh from that one.

Another slice of humor I like to throw in every once in a while to make my mom laugh is to tell her that she's super-hot because thanks to her InterStim implant, she has a "bun" of steel. We both chuckle at that one with tongue-in-cheek. And it's always amusing when my Mom's InterStim device will set off the security alarm at a big box or retail store. If she walks too close to the security barrier, it will most likely start to beep. You have to be able to laugh at yourself and not take anything too seriously. Life is too short to over-stress yourself with worries, anxiety and the unknown. If you can find the silver lining and humor in each situation you go through, having an InterStim implant will be a piece of cake. And to wrap it up, always refer to this quote, again from the marvelous Mark Twain, "Humor is the great thing, the saving thing after all. The minute it crops up, all our anxiety yielded, all our irritations, and resentments flit away, and a sunny spirit takes their place." Take this quote with you and you will not go wrong, no matter what challenges you may encounter.

What I Think

Top 10 things everyone should know about IC from an IC Patient Advocate's Experience and Perspective:

1. *You* have IC, IC <u>does not</u> have you. This is extremely important when dealing with the daily ups and downs of Interstitial Cystitis. Don't let your life come to a halt. Learn how to help yourself and take control of your disease. Do not let your disease control you.

2. Don't ever take no for an answer when your health is at stake. If the admitting nurse at the ER says to your patient advocate that he or she cannot come back to the room with you, simply tell the nurse or medical assistant that if your patient advocate isn't allowed to go back, you (the patient there seeking help) won't be going back. This has yet to stop anyone from letting me (the patient advocate) go back in the ER room or back at any appointment with my mom (the patient).

3. Ask for help. No one can help you if they don't know something is wrong in the first place.

4. Laugh. Having a sense of humor and being able to not only laugh at awkward situations, possibly inappropriate topics and

through stressful times, but also at yourself, will help you survive the most painful episodes of IC.

5. Accept your limitations. Know when to let someone else help you, know when to accept help, know when to agree that you *can't* do something. Allow yourself to rest when needed. Give yourself a break. This disease is no cakewalk.

6. Educate others. Too many people still do not have any idea what IC is, what it does, how it effects someone's health and life, the pain it causes, etc. Find ways to explain it to others in layman's terms so that they can understand what your disease is about. The more people who know, the better off you will be and the more help and comfort you will be offered.

7. Do not be afraid to fight the insurance companies if they initially turn you down for a medication, procedure or doctor you have been referred to. Even if they turn you down a second time, keep fighting. You *can* win. We have won several battles all due to persistence that were predetermined "impossible" by various professionals in the medical field.

8. Do your research. Doctors often prescribe drugs without having the time or resources to check if they will interact with the patient's current medications, medical condition, health history, etc. It is crucial to your own well being to read all of the drug's ingredients, side effects, check your drug interactions, etc. You will usually know after a few key points if it is a drug worth trying, if it's okay to take, etc. Ask your pharmacist if they can do a drug interaction report for you to double check everything and keep a copy in your medical files for future reference.

9. Make yourself stay positive. It is too easy when dealing with BPS/IC to allow you to sink into a deep hole of depression, self-pity, and see everything in a negative light. Remain focused on the positive things in your life. Find people who are encouraging and supportive, criticism you do not need. What are the activities that give you joy, provide healthy distraction and make dealing with IC just a little less stressful, painful and frustrating.

10. Do not ignore your pain. Treat it, address it, do whatever it takes to get rid of your pain so that you are not suffering. This can start to wear you out, take up time, become exhausting, possibly become annoying because it may happen frequently, but no matter what, do what you have to do to get your pain to take a hike. As Dr. Davis likes to state, "No one ever won any awards for staying in pain". You already have IC, you already have enough to deal with and daily struggles to get through. Find a solution, discover different coping tools, experiment with relaxation techniques, research different medications, talk to your doctor about your options and explore what works best for you. But above all else, do not even try to ignore your pain and not address it. It will eat you alive, but only if you let it.

3. Carole, age 61
Bethany's Mom: My BPS/IC Journey

I am a 61 year-old, married, mother of two adult children, my daughter, is 29 and son, 24 years old. I am living and dealing with IC since diagnosed eight years ago. I have had health complications most of my life so being diagnosed with IC was a nuisance, but not a complete shock. I had been down this road before in respect to additional medical appointments, surgeries, procedures, prescriptions, insurance battles and anything else that came into play from major health issues.

I have never smoked, drink alcohol only socially, and not very much when I do. I stay active with friends and family and I love to travel. My career as an elementary school librarian means the school year never really ends. As with my other health issues I have refused to let my IC control my life.

I do not feel that I can begin telling my Interstitial Cystitis story without giving some basic and relevant medical history and incidents that started at a very young age for me. I unfortunately started my period when I was eleven years old and my menstrual cycles were always heavy and extremely painful. I cannot remember a time since I began my period that I wasn't in tons of discomfort and pain.

I was not aware that anything was physically wrong and accepted my monthly pelvic pain as what happens to some a time of menstruation. After I was married. I found sex to be extremely painful and not at all enjoyable as it should have been. It took me forever to find a doctor that would sincerely listen to me and take my pain and concerns seriously. As a newlywed, I was only viewed as a new bride who was nervous and uptight about sex. I was told a variety of non-helpful tips such as "Just relax, don't get uptight. You'll get the hang of it"; "It will be fine, you're just nervous"; I had one doctor say the following, "Go home, have a stiff drink and take a Valium." I even had one gynecologist prescribe heavy fertility drugs without my knowledge or consent.

Along with Interstitial Cystitis, I battle a handful of additional health complications and conditions at the same time. I am currently taking prescriptions for hormone replacement, depression, acid reflux, chronic migraine headaches, cholesterol, a minor heart murmur, allergies and anxiety. My current medicine regime includes: Allegra, Elmiron (instillations), Zoloft, Wellbutrin, (prescribed by my Primary physician for depression and anxiety) Prilosec, Flexerial, Estrace, Klonopin, Benedryl, and Fiorinal with codeine. My vitamins include Citracal (Calcium and D), Vitamin B, and a Women's Metabolism One-A-Day vitamin supplement.

I have a small variety of painkillers that I take for my Interstitial Cystitis. These include Pyridium (prescribed by my urologist for bladder pain) and morphine (prescribed by the pain management specialist.) Pyridium is likely the most helpful drug that I have taken for IC. It calms the pain down much faster then other drugs I have and it turns my pee a lovely shade of bright orange! Only a few anxieties about the drugs – Pyridium makes me as dry as the Sahara desert, it also turns my pee bright orange and is quite a shocker when I haven't taken it in a while. I tried and stopped taking Lyrica (a drug for neurogenic pain) because I started to gain extreme weight and refused to go that far. When my bladder pain gets to be too excruciating, I take morphine, which occasionally will cause a rebound headache. My only drug allergies include Demerol and Gadolinium (the MRI dye).

One of my biggest challenges with medication is that although I look small, in bone structure and weight, I have an extremely high tolerance to drugs. It has been very frustrating when doctors do not believe me when I am still walking and talking without problems after 10mg of morphine. Some of the other drugs I have tried for my IC included Lyrica for the neurogenic pain, but also, an antispasmodic for the bladder, that is to calm the bladder down as Pyridium does, also have tried Elavil, Neurontin, and Sanctura.

Finally, I saw a gynecologist whom after just one simple pelvic exam, discovered a huge tumor located in my vaginal canal. After this initial appointment, he did a laparoscopy and found out from doing that very minor but crucial procedure that I was covered in endometriosis. This painful and devastating diagnosis led to my complete hysterectomy in 1979 at the ripe age of 28. I was a newly married, never been pregnant, and now infertile.

Unfortunately, even after the hysterectomy procedure, sex was painful and uncomfortable for me. Although my periods and painful cramping were gone, I was still extremely prone to urinary tract infections. I never had the frequency/urgency symptom, but I had urinary retention most of my life, never realizing that my ability to hold my pee for hours on end was unusual. I am 98% positive that my IC woke up at the time of my hysterectomy. Back then, a hysterectomy was performed using an open incision and not with a laparoscope through the belly button. My insides were moved around, removed, rearranged and then thrown back in, creating some kind of chaos along with the wonderful souvenir of adhesions resulting from scar tissue. I feel strongly that this particular surgery could definitely have been the trigger to start the rumblings of BPS/IC; perhaps something was nicked accidentally or the adhesions started to slowly wrap around my poor tiny bladder, causing it to eventually react and rebel.

After the hysterectomy I had a five-day stay in the hospital; back in those days you were actually allowed to recover in the hospital after major surgery for more than eight hours. I had what is called an indwelling latex catheter the direct contact with latex could have also set up the start of my IC symptoms. The fact is that many IC patients are extremely sensitive to latex. It is commonly used in all medical environments.

I first went to see an urologist who knew IC well in 2003. I was referred to him from my primary care physician as a result of having several subsequent painful bladder infections and there were continuous traces of blood found in my urine that no antibiotic would cure. My initial symptoms did not lineup with a typical IC patient. I had mild urinary retention and frequently what I thought to be bladder infections. But I did not have any urgency or frequency problems, I did not have pelvic pain, burning sensations, essentially nothing BPS/IC patient typically describes when seeking out an urologist.

After his initial exam, evaluation of my current physical condition and preliminary questions, the doctor's initial diagnosis, because of the consistent traces of blood in my urine, was that I most likely had some form of cancer in the bladder or possibly elsewhere. He ordered a cystoscopy and after much anxiety and overcoming nerves, I went to the hospital to see what was going on with my bladder. The procedure went well and afterwards I received the infamous bladder pictures, revealing that I definitely had an angry, inflamed bladder and that Interstitial Cystitis was the cause.

After this initial cystoscopy, the pain started to surface and truly presented itself. I started to have extremely uncomfortable pelvic pain, urethral burning, bladder spasms and horrible complications with getting my bladder to release when I tried to go to the bathroom. Unlike the majority of IC patients, my primary symptom and complication with IC has been urinary retention. This means I need to void and have the urge but cannot release the urine that continues to be produced by my kidneys and stored in my bladder that becomes more and more distended. As the pain grows the only way for me to have relief is catheterization.

The problem started as something I could handle but quickly moved from annoying, to awful, to severe bladder pain. I tried many a warm bath, warm baths with Epson salts, relaxation techniques, once a week visits to the IC clinic where I received lidocaine/sodium bicarbonate and Elmiron instillation treatments, and unfortunately, frequent trips to the emergency room so they could handle draining my bladder, administer a rescue treatment (lidocaine/sodium bicarbonate and give some kind of painkiller (usually morphine worked best for me) and then send me home. I consistently had to deal with the frustrating circumstances of doctors and nurses not knowing what IC even was, the horrifying and unreal accusation of drug seeking, not believing I could hold a 1000+ ccs of urine in my bladder, dealing with nurses that didn't have a clue of how to administer the "Rescue" treatment and being treated as what I felt a common criminal for a chronic disease that I was still trying to understand.

After too many trips to the ER, my daughter and I created a "Rescue Card" for fellow IC patients to carry with them to present to ER nurses and doctors to receive the appropriate and accurate treatment they needed when in severe pain.

Bladder Pain Syndrome/Interstitial Cystitis (BPS/IC)
Edward L. Davis, MD – 412 W Caroll Ave. Suite 200 – Glendora, CA 91741
(626) 914-3921

Emergency Rescue Procedure:
- Soak baby, plastic, self-lubricating catheter according to directions. AstraTech (1-3 Min) to activate coated exterior film.
- Clean area around opening of the bladder. (Urethral area)
- For comfort, apply lidocaine jelly to urethral area.
- Insert catheter slowly through the urethral opening only until urine comes out.
  Note: For a woman, the urethra is 1 to 1 ½ inches long – May have to cough to start flow of urine.
- Drain urine until bladder is empty.
- Measure about of urine removed (in CCs).
- Test and send to lab for Culture and Sensitivity for red blood cells, nitrites, etc.
- Instill lidocaine rescue through the catheter into the bladder.

Rescue mix:
- 25 CCs of 1 or 2% sterile lidocaine plus 10ccs of sterile sodium bicarbonate.
- Have patient gently roll from side to side to medicate the bladder.

At Home:
- Bicarbonate of soda bath in warm water. Bed rest. Covered icepack to urethral area.

Doctor_____ Date_____

I will be very blunt, I HATE having Interstitial Cystitis. I don't look sick, I can still put on a smile, but NO ONE truly knows or even understands when they look at me how much pain I am in; no one knows what I go through at home, with doctors, with drugs, and with the IC symptoms.

My greatest frustration is that neither the medical establishment nor the public   knows what the IC disease is and how the negative impact of the symptoms escalates. If I had cancer, no one would have a second thought as to how I was feeling, dealing with my job, how I was able to get up every day, etc. I am angry that IC is labeled chronic and that I will have to deal with this disease the rest of my life. The pain that I live with on a daily basis has become second nature and is often unbearable. It can range from throbbing pain, sometimes if feels like there's a hot poker up my urethra, and when I go to the bathroom there is definitely some sort of muscular reaction that feels like my bladder is being squeezed and causes pain and burning *almost* every time I urinate. On the medical pain scale of 1-10, I personally function almost daily at a 4, which is described as moderate pain. If not a 4, I can usually survive at a 5 that is basically described as you should be lying down or sitting with ice; but instead I have to work. I do not have a choice at the moment due to hard economic times and although my job as an elementary school librarian has me sitting the majority of the work day, I also have books to re-shelve on a daily basis, materials to look up, students to assist and chores to keep up for my daily responsibilities.

BPS/IC flares, for me, do not have a rhyme or a reason. I can easily have two to three IC flares a month, sometimes one a month, and on very rare occasions, not at all in a thirty day period. What sets a flare off one time, mostly likely will not be the cause of the next one. My bladder flares are extremely painful and my emotions usually go for a roller coaster ride. They can drag me into severe depression; bring me to tears without much provocation, and overall create a real sensitivity to everything. With IC, I feel that my emotions are on overdrive, sensitivity-wise. I am also fatigued all the time. My body and bladder feel constantly at war with each other. The combination of pain, stress, drugs and the fight to work through it, make me exhausted.

I also find that I am not able to push through the pain and fatigue like I used to. I don't like to admit it, but age is most likely a factor for this. I almost always sleep with an ice pack, sleep more elevated due to acid reflux, and the urge to pee (which I gladly accept from not being able to pee before getting my InterStim an electronic, implanted device that stimulates the sacral nerve and sends a signal to my bladder to void) is usually the only thing that wakes me up these days. Before I had my InterStim implant, I was getting up 3-4 times a night to either pee or sit on the toilet, hoping I would pee (the urge was there, but the urinary retention would not allow my bladder to release anything). Now, after having the InterStim implant for over 2 years, I might get up one time a night, but not always.

When I occasionally get a true bladder infection, I almost always have to have my urine sample sent out to be cultured so the right antibiotic can be prescribed to get rid of it, otherwise the infection may linger for weeks on end and only add to my discomfort and pain level. A bladder infection can add to the inflammation of IC and increase the bladder pain.

Whenever and for whatever reason and IC flare happens, I usually come home from work in the afternoon, put an ice pack to my perineum to calm the burning in my bladder down, take a painkiller and then a nap usually follows. This routine typically helps my bladder pain subside for a few hours, but once I have to go to the bathroom again, my bladder spasms, the pain spikes, and the cycle repeat itself. It is exhausting. Let me say they stress definitely has a huge role in causing an IC pain to escalate. We are under extreme financial burdens at home along with the pressure of high demands from my boss and work.

Since I was diagnosed with IC, I have been on a strict regime using ice packs almost every afternoon and night applied to my crotch area, plus Allegra, Zoloft, and a painkiller. One of the handiest tools and pain relieving aides I have come across has been small ice gel packs that freeze sold. These are usually at Target; I believe they are usually used for your kid's lunch packs. They are small, convenient, durable, and most of them have lasted me for years. Any new IC patient will quickly learn that "Ice is your friend!"

I tried was Dimethyl Sulfoxide (DMSO), which made me smell like a garlic farm once a week. It was painful, only provided temporarily relief and was an extremely unpleasant experience and my IC symptoms continued along with my severe urinary retention.

Eventually I was diagnosed with a neurogenic bladder, meaning that my bladder does not respond to my brain's signals that it needs to release urine. In response to my unusual symptoms and unresponsive treatment attempts, my urologist had mentioned with a hesitant recommendation that I might try an InterStim, which could possibly help alleviate my urinary retention through electronic stimulation. At first I was scared of the prospect of an InterStim, mainly due to the fact that all I found were negative reviews, horror stories, and tales of thumping, and pulsating, etc. as the sensations from the implant that stimulates the sacral nerve. Unfortunately, by my insurance ruled out the urologist as the surgeon to perform the InterStim surgery, and I had to find another resource, which turned out to be the Pain Management route.

I was referred to the Rehabilitation Institute in where I could receive further help and treatment for my debilitating migraine headaches. It was determined after an MRI and several tests, that I had spinal stenosis in the C4, C5 of my spine. Since then, 3-4 times a year I have a cervical epidural done (they last approximately 3 months). The spinal stenosis is still there, but epidurals have most definitely helped my migraine headache intensity and frequency.

While being treated by the doctors at PRI, I also started to receive treatment to address my chronic pain from IC. This was where my journey to getting my InterStim implant began. After much deliberation, meeting with Medtronic patient reps, doctor's appointments, questions and research, in April of 2009, I did the trial surgery for the InterStim and it worked almost like magic.

The trial period for the InterStim is mandatory to see if the device will indeed help the patient and involved the small device being partially inserted into my right buttock area and a battery pack being attached to my waist for three to four days. I was surprised and thrilled with the almost immediate ability to go to the bathroom and actually pee! The trial was deemed a total success and I underwent surgery to have the Medtronic's InterStim permanently implanted. In my opinion, it has worked miracles. It is such a relief that I can actually empty my bladder when I go to the bathroom. I am still doing at-home Elmiron instillation treatments twice a week with the help of my daughter and it definitely helps keep my bladder and IC at bay. Almost exactly one year later I had to have the InterStim repositioned because it had come too close to the surface and it was beginning to become extremely uncomfortable.

Initially, I started to drain the urine from my bladder with the use of catheterizations on my own at home due to the horrible retention I was dealing with and so I could avoid going to the emergency room as often; eventually we started doing rescue treatments and Elmiron instillations at home in addition to just draining my bladder to cut down on doctor appointments, time, money, and of course cut out frequent trips to the ER.

Currently, with my daughter's help, I do 2-3 Elmiron instillations a week from the comfort of our home. To some this may appear strange, extreme or unnecessary, but trust me when I say that finally accepting the responsibility of doing rescues and Elmiron treatments on my own at home has been both a blessing and a lifesaver. We have invested in several inexpensive tools to make the instillation process flow as smoothly as possible. We lay a trash bag and a beach towel down on the bed and the gather sanitary wipes, a catheter (plastic not latex) a small plastic bowl, lidocaine jelly, and a syringe that has sterile lidocaine and sterile sodium bicarbonate mix.

The lidocaine is to temporally numb my bladder and the sodium bicarbonate neutralizes the acid being produced urine so tha the Elmiron will not have to fight as much urine acidity. The Elmiron used is directed as to amount by the urologist and is mixed with sterile sodium chloride. The reason for this procedure has two points: (1) direct application of Elmiron coats the bladder wall to protect it from urine (2) the thought that lidocaine even in small amounts may give relief by numbing the bladder nerves. When I am finished with the catheterization it's off to sit with an ice pack on my crotch.

Since being diagnosed with IC, I have become keenly aware of my diet and its affects on my body. I also have horrible acid reflex, so if foods don't affect my bladder, there's a good chance they're going to cause my acid reflex to flare up. My food sensitivities defined as anything that causes bladder pain, burning, a flare or anything of the sort include: orange juice, grapefruit, anything citrus or acidic is out of the question, anything spicy, processed meats and most fast food options. I do enjoy drinking soft drinks and have discovered that I can have Coke Cola brand in moderation but absolutely NO Pepsi products due to the potassium they put in their drinks.

Since being diagnosed with IC, I have definitely increased my bottled water consumption; I drink nothing but Arrowhead (spring water source) brand. After one of the IC support group meetings where different types and brands of bottled water was tested, Arrowhead was found to be the most IC friendly, so it's been nothing but Arrowhead bottled water since. I have definitely learned what particular or types of foods and drinks affect my bladder and body overall, and the one food that I have discovered I am allergic to and makes my mouth break out into sores whenever I eat them are walnuts. This makes me very sad because I used to be able to eat them without any problem and I cannot seem to find any source to explain this allergy. Safe IC foods for me include chicken, beef (steak, roast, etc.), fresh fish, vegetables, fruit, salad, coke products (in moderation), sweet wine (red or white), breads, chocolate and most desserts.

I have not let IC limit my life in very many ways including traveling. I love to travel and have dragged my pharmacy and rescue treatment supplies on Girl Scout trips, camping outings, to Canada on a family trip and I have even had the fine traveling experience of having an ice pack delivered to me by room service at the Park Plaza Hotel in London, England (You have to keep a great sense of humor when getting through each day with IC)!! I do have to pack like a pharmacy when I travel and wherever I go I carry an emergency kit which includes painkiller, catheter, rescue treatment supplies, my IC rescue card, and anything else I may need at the moment to effectively treat my bladder. Another small obstacle when traveling is I can no longer go through the medical detectors due to my InterStim implant. I carry an official Medtronic card that states what I have and the instructions for whoever may need them.

My strongest ally from the moment I was diagnosed has been my daughter, from monitoring doctor's appointments, to the many ER crises of the past, and supporting home instillation treatments, she has been there. She's accompanied me to almost every doctor's visit since we discovered I had Interstitial Cystitis, has taken the time to educate her herself, been my advocate; when we go to the ER, they put her to work. She educates others, is my biggest defender, stands up for me, gets me what I need, makes sure I am fully prepared with supplies, ice, relaxation tools, etc. My daughter helps me at least 3-4 times a week re-shelve the books in my library and we have calculated that we re-shelve an average of 150-200 books on a daily basis. Without her help in re-shelving the primary books on the very low shelves, I would not be able to handle my job while dealing with my IC. I am blessed.

I have to accept that my young son is not interested in being educated about BPS/IC. My husband and I do not have a very positive or close relationship, but this was not caused by the IC diagnosis or having the disease itself. I do know, however, from different things he has said and from what others have told me that he understands more about my disease and my pain than he lets on. He does defend me when others try and say something about my inactivity, pain, etc. He is very willing to get ice for me, something to drink and help make me comfortable, etc. Our relationship not being that great has nothing to do with my IC.

When I think back to the number of doctors and ER visits for my Mother, for what we thought were many a bladder infection, I know almost without a doubt, that she had IC. On family trips I can remember having to constantly find bathrooms for her, taking her to the emergency room for what we thought were bladder infections.

I feel like I have 90% control of my life but that my BPS/IC still has 10% and that puts me in my place and makes me catch my breath every once in a while. Relaxation items and coping tools that I found do improve my quality of life and help reduce pain have been warm/hot baths, massages, sitting in the spa, spending time with my dog and finding different activities to do that I enjoy that will help distract me from thinking about my pain and disease. Other changes I have made include not doing any heavy lifting, not doing heavy housework and accepting that there are certain things I cannot (and most importantly should not) do with my bladder disease. My IC has definitely altered my ability to perform certain everyday activities. Thankfully my daughter constantly reminds me to limit myself and helps me do things that I should and sometimes cannot do anymore.

Another huge coping tool that has helped me in many different ways is my faith. I believe strongly in God, that He has a plan for me and that everything happens for a reason; but I am so angry, frustrated, and tired of having this painful and misunderstood disease. I get so aggravated when someone who knows I have this disease asks me, "Haven't you gotten rid of that thing (IC) yet?" or others who have the nerve to say "You don't look sick."

There are multiple triggers that will set my IC off and my bladder into a flare with very little effort. Negative factors include stress, extreme emotional situations, work, pressure by my boss and teachers at the school where I work, money pressures and a very stressful home life. My husband has been unemployed for several years and the weight of all the household and personal finances are solely on the shoulders of my daughter and me.

As a person living with a chronic disease, especially one as unknown and misunderstood as Interstitial Cystitis, you are going to have to stand up for yourself, probably more than you may be comfortable with. It will be to your extreme benefit to have someone become your personal patient advocate. This is someone you trust to go with you to appointments, help you through the emotional ups and downs of IC, help you through the painful flares, listen to the doctors, surgeons, nurses, medical assistants and office staff, take notes and hear details and instructions that you may miss because of your pain or frustration. It is also smart to have a second set of ears and eyes to cover all bases.

Always remember that you are not alone. There are, in my opinion, thousands upon thousands of individuals living with this painful and frustrating condition. I encourage you to use the support networks, support groups, and resources that are available.

Information about Interstitial Cystitis/Bladder Pain Syndrome needs to spread as much as possible because there are many more individuals out there who have IC and are not aware. They do not understand why they are suffering. The more aware people become of Interstitial Cystitis, the more help, research, and fight for a cure there will be.

When you are feeling frustrated, confused, in pain, and not knowing where to turn next, repeat this quote to yourself, "I have IC; IC does not have me."

My Top 10 list for what every patient dealing with IC should know and follow:

What I Think
1. Don't ignore symptoms – Sexual pain, microscopic blood in your urine, constant bladder infections, don't let the medical community write you off, keep fighting and searching for a doctor with knowledge and one that will listen to your needs, feelings, symptoms, etc. and most importantly, a doctor who will *believe* you.

2. It is a must to develop a hard spine and thick skin. You have to stand up for yourself though the tough times. Learn to say no when your health is at stake.

3. Find yourself an advocate. Even after you get an advocate, get a dog.

4. Educate yourself. Seek information wherever you can find it. Internet (i.e. IC Network, icaction.com), medical journals, research, etc. The more you know and soak in, the more you will learn how to live and conquer IC.

5. Laugh. Have a sense of humor. If you don't have one, get one quick. Laughter has helped my daughter and I through some tough and painful episodes, awkward situations and stressful times. Make yourself laugh. Finding humor in things that you never found funny or amusing before will be one of your best friends though your IC journey.

6. Seek the comfort and company of others who have IC. They will be your biggest supporters, sympathizers, strongest shoulders to cry on and the ones who truly understand what you're going through, how to deal with it, and advice you can actually use instead of being offended by truths.

7. Do not EVER let anyone tell you that the pain is not real. Sexual pain, pain when you go to the bathroom, aching and throbbing pain, etc. The pain is REAL. You have to be willing to do something about it. Whether it is seeking the comfort of ice, a hot bath, taking painkiller, relaxation techniques, etc. You need to be willing to help yourself. Learn how to help yourself and then force yourself to do it.

8. As painful and annoying as it is, watch your diet. You can ignore what you eat and drink, but eventually it will catch up to you and then eventually down to your bladder. Don't stop living and enjoying what you like, but remember to take certain trigger foods or beverages in moderation if you must have them.

9. Always be prepared no matter where you are, where you go or whom you're with. Whether it's for an overnight in the mountains, on a family camping trip or off in Europe for 2 weeks, take your supplies, drugs, Rx script, doctor's notes, medical letters, Rescue Card, doctor's instructions, medical insurance information, etc. Put yourself first and accept the fact that this disease cannot be ignored unless you're looking for painful consequences.

10. Be willing to seek out and fight for solutions that work for you. Be willing to take risks, try new avenues; whatever it takes that might help improve your quality of life. If I had listened to everyone about the InterStim and gone with their opinions, I would have never even tried the InterStim implant. It is truly one of the best decisions I have ever made for myself and without it, I would be truly miserable and my level of daily discomfort from IC would be tenfold from what it is now. As a person living with IC, one must remember that every single patient is completely different. Every person will react differently to different medications, treatments, surgeries, etc. You *have* to be willing to go out on a limb and find what works best for *you*.

4. Joan, age 52
BPS/IC: All in the Family

Background

My Name is Joan, and I am 52 years old. My husband and I have jointly lived one hundred and nine years with our five children. They range in age from twenty-seven to thirteen.

I begin my story with the introduction of my children because as their Mom, I continued to make multiple bathroom visits just as I had needed to do during my growing up years. My dad and Mom made family vacation car trips an adventure of frequent restroom stops for me. For two of my five children, I followed my childhood pattern of planning any away from home outing armed with the knowledge that there would be multiple pee stops. I truly believed that my other three children had the urinary problems because they never seemed to need to go. But as it was discovered my eldest and youngest share my IC diagnosis.

In my teenage and young adult years I often had sharp pelvic pain and from time to time the pelvic misery was a dull thudding pain sensation. It made sense to me then that the problem was my uterus. I never thought about the bladder or the urethra as source.

With my marriage came the realization that sexual intercourse was painful. The search for a cause led me to ten gynecologists. I was diagnosed with Pelvic Inflammatory Disease (PID) and the resolution was supposed to be found in lots of Ibuprofen (Motrin) and hot baths. For me, this management helped. What added to my confusion was that when the pelvic pain was bad and I felt it would never end, it would suddenly subside. Years would go by before I made connections to my pelvic pain increasing before my period; all I knew was that the pain cycle went on and on. This was my life, I made the most and best of it.

Then came the physicians who thought that perhaps the reason for this merry-go-round of pelvic pain was caused by bladder infections. I was given antibiotics and sent on my way. To this day I do not recall any physician sending my urine to a lab for a culture. I didn't know to ask if they checked if I had a true infection. All I wanted was not to hurt.

In 1993 vulvar pain came into my life and the specialist whose answer for me was urethral dilations. I think it made the pain worse. But desperate times call for desperate measures, and that was me.

About eight years ago came the revelation that if all the doctors I had seen over the years in my search for the cause of my pelvic and vulvar pain had not been able to give me an answer as to why; chances were they just didn't know.

One physician told me, "Oh, you don't want that (IC), get rid of it," I knew it was up to me to find out what was pushing my life in such a negative direction. I had to keep looking.

Then a miracle, a kidney stones showed up on an x-ray. Those tiny stones were tangible evidence that could be dealt with by an urologist. In all those doctor visits the specialty of urology never came up. I was diagnosed with IC in 1999 because of scoping my bladder for those kidney stones. Finally I could put a definite name to the reason for my pelvic pain. The knowledge that I had IC took me from thinking I was neurotic and dismissing my pain, to appreciating that I had a lot to learn.

When my seventeen-year-old daughter was diagnosed with IC and six months later my five-year-old son was also formally diagnosed, I remembered their infant years. Of my five children my oldest daughter and youngest son were the two that always had wet diapers and potty training was a nightmare. With the diagnosis of IC so much of our lives now made sense.

Since we discovered that we shared the symptom patterns of IC, I knew they were watching how I handled my own recovery. I was now a role model for how to handle a chronic disease. I had to learn how to help them by educating myself.

I knew I needed to gather as much information as possible so that I could begin to sort through what symptom relief solutions work for me and might help my children. One of the best decisions I made was to attend the Interstitial Cystitis Associations (ICA) seminar in Florida followed by an ICA convention in Minnesota. I began to build my library of IC focused books. And in 2001, I found the IC support group. I began to attend and become involved in both learning and sharing information about the syndrome that is IC. I was able to take greater control with the personal assessment of IC information and how it related to our lives.

Becoming informed makes all the difference, as illustrated by an event in my daughter's life before I was aware that children could have IC. When my daughter was in the fifth grade the class project was to learn how to budget money. Students were to pay rent for their school desk as a part of their expenses; also each restroom visit had a fee. Because of her urinary frequency she ran out of money and lost her desk and had to sit on the floor. This hurtful event was caused by the lack of information and understanding. On the reverse side, my young son has returned to school each year to teachers who I have informed about his special needs. A night and day difference in the school experience because of my education of what to expect with his IC symptoms.

My personal food and allergy discoveries are reflected in both my children. For me the allergic response to the antibiotic tetracycline and sulfa medication is throat swelling. This throat tightening and inability to breathe also happens to my daughter when the vegetable, asparagus, even touches her plate. I vividly remember a call to the paramedics that was aided with my giving her the antihistamine, Benadryl. I have learned about genetic links from my children.

For us, definitely, preservatives and monosodium glutamate (MSG) cause bladder and pelvic distress. As an example, I eat all fresh vegetables and fruit with the exception of plums and walnuts; I must be sensitive to these two foods because my throat gets sore.

About five years ago I became a patient advocate in the urology office IC Clinic. I have never smoke, had any coffee, tea with caffeine, or alcohol, including wine or beer, as part of my life. After discussions with many IC patients I recognize and appreciate how difficult it is to modify these choices even when you know the rationale is to make BPS/IC symptoms less likely to occur.

I have listened to patient statements that their drink choices make no difference in their IC symptoms. I think they do. I have diabetes and I am controlled with oral medication and diet. I can drink the cola brand of Diet Coke with no bladder reaction, but if I drink the brand Diet Pepsi pelvic pain comes. I discovered that Pepsi has potassium and Diet Coke does not and that must make the difference in reactions for me. Caffeine acts on me, as is reported by most, with more trips to void. I'm fortunate and have ducked the pelvic pain bullet with this one. Directly after drinking a cola I drink sixteen ounces of spring water of the southern California brands, Arrowhead, Crystal Geyer or the brand called Evian, because it has minerals; this mean a lower acid content (pH) than the reverse osmosis products such as Aquafina, Dasani, or any bottled water labeled "drinking."

For most of the week we have nine dietary plans to consider. As an example I deal with diabetes and the fresh fruits and vegetables balance well with the IC. A low acid diet, limiting dyes, preservative, and going mainly organic for our choices takes the entire family's health into account. Due to my diabetes, my need is to reduce quantity of the starch items such as rice and potatoes, which are the corner stone of the IC diet.

I am a believer that our food is the major source of the chemicals we put in our bodies. What we choose to eat and drink makes a huge difference in maintaining good health. When I prepare the meals I always consider our needed dietary adjustments. I cook mostly using fresh not preserved. I have often said that before a food is dismissed from the diet the source, i.e. organic, the way it is prepared, i.e. baked tomatoes instead of raw, and amount of consumed should be considered before it is thrown out of a diet as not being tolerated.

The extra money spent on purchasing organic foods, Bristol Farms and time finding good sources of prepared meals, such as Trader Joes has been worth it because it is less time and money spent fighting IC flares and doctor visits.

When it comes to restaurants I find that more and more of the chains are learning that customers want choices based on being nutritious rather than taste alone. Again we are fortunate to have a family chain of "In and Out Burger." That keeps it menus simple and the food choices freshly made.

I know my allergy ranges from medications such as tetracycline and all sulfa-based drugs. I know that monosodium glutamate (MSG) has the same affect on me as eating walnuts; my throat gets sore. I have learned to read my body's messages.

My main medication for IC remains Elmiron. I now take 200mg a day, one in the morning and one in the evening. Zyrtec is the antihistamine that I take before bedtime to keep the environmental allergies quieted down. I do not know what studies have been done but for me allergies are a big part of my bladder and vulvar pain control. Calcium citrate with D is part of my health regimen. My main reason for the addition of calcium citrate to my medication list is the suggestion of the Vulvar Pain organization; for me this combination works well.

When you have five children, I did my share of lifting. Along my educational way I discovered that asking for help with the heavy lifting was smart. We all have to learn where our boundaries are. As other examples to keep me fit; running and aerobics have been replaced with walking and aerobics in a pool. Low impact has become more than a phrase to me.

There is much to be said for the healing act of sleeping. My bedtime is between ten and eleven o'clock, and because I have learned to live the changes that needed to made, I no longer take my middle of the night walks to the bathroom. Sleeping through to six thirty in the morning is the blessing of my much-improved life.

A large part of my support has been my husband. There were long rough patches when I didn't understand why my pelvic region and vulva were so painful and the frustration spilled over into our marriage. We need to pull together because in our house we are a large family and it is multigenerational. For the past several years and for the foreseeable future we have a busy household with my mother-in-law and father-in-law, my oldest daughter, son-in-law, their new baby, and our two sons. My aim was to educate most of my family members. They need to understand the reasons for the choices we have to make because of the need to control IC symptoms, in addition to multiple other individual dietary needs.

Difficult times came for me when I tried to explain the nature of IC with my attempts to share with my mother-in-law; how we needed to work together so that IC was taken into account. Most of my family members understand that any chronic condition means ongoing up keep, IC is no different, in my opinion. My mother-in-law is in her mid-seventies and does not open her mind to many changes. This reminds me of the majority of the physicians I have asked for help over the years. In my experience, too many times a physician would not admit to not understanding the reason for my distress and deny there was a problem; perhaps my mother-in-law's outlook is the same. I have decided you cannot win them all.

I have come a long way from wondering where to turn for help. The anger caused by pain and frustration has changed into self-reliance to make decisions based on solid information. Life has its trials, errors, and hard times; I encourage you to find the support you need so that you can again find joy.

What I Think:
1. All childhood repetitive experiences are not always "normal." My parents made great allowances to deal with my frequent bathroom stops.

2. If sexual intercourse is painful, there is a problem.

3. If you have bladder infection symptoms, such as increased urge, frequency, burning or pain or urination, and even a tiny amount of blood is found in your urine, a sample needs to be sent to the lab to check for bacteria. Differences in dealing with an IC flare and Urinary tract Infection (UTI) must be taken in to account.

4. Vulvar pain and IC pain are when nerves are hyper-activated.

5. Be prepared to search for a physician who understands IC. This situation of lack of awareness is improving, but there is still a less than perfect system of identification and treatment.

6. The Interstitial Cystitis Association (ICA) has a wealth of good information. It is up to the individual to decide when the information can guide them.

7. I think that IC can be passed from generation to generation, just like sensitivities and allergies.

8. Diet changes are a key to IC control. Think organic and homegrown and homemade.

9. Pharmaceutical medication in our treatment should not be discounted just as the homeopathic or herbal methods should not be embraced without the appreciation that they are all chemicals.

10. Take your body's message seriously. Ask for help, and learn to say no.

5. Laura, age 27
I'm Joan's Daughter and Daniel is My Brother

Background
Laura is 27 years old, born and raised in Southern California. The eldest of five, two brothers and three sisters, married for six years. She is planning on having a family. Her career choice is surgical nurse. Mother and youngest brother have BPS/IC.

Laura's Story

My earliest recollections are tied in with the need to go to the bathroom to pee, sometimes more than fifteen times a day. I knew that carbonated drinks and fast foods made the need to void even greater. Fruit juices brought on a sensation of burning as I voided. These are my childhood remembrances when someone talks about IC.

The family process was for me to use the bathroom before we left the house because everyone knew I would have to go again just as the key was turned in the ignition. As a child a great frustration for my family and me, were the wait lines at Disneyland. I had to deal with losing our place in line because of a restroom trip. The stress of peeing in strange surroundings, with joys of Disneyland just outside the door was a lot for a youngster to accept.

When I think back to grade school there are hurtful events tied to the need to pee. In the fifth grade our class was ready to go on a field trip; everyone was told to go to the restroom, and I did. We arrived at the destination and I had to go again. My Mom was there as a chaperone and she approached the teacher about another trip to the restroom. The first response by the teacher was, "no." I know if my Mom had not been there the teacher would not have let me go. In the fifth grade there was class trip to a magnificent music hall. On that trip, when my Mother said we needed to return to the restroom; the teacher said there were no restrooms available. The same teacher had a lesson about how to budget money. She took away my desk because I spent my budgeted money on going to the toilet. To this day a hurtful aspect of my memories of grade school is wondering why teachers would not believe a youngster in distress. Thank goodness my Mom was often there to protect me.

Vacations would produce their own special problems. I remember a flight to Wisconsin. The flight attendant told my Mom that I went too often to lavatory and not to go again during the flight.

Because my Mother also had the same urinary urge and frequency cycle we more often than not went together. It was my Dad who had the patience to make the stops. For that I will always be grateful.

When I was thirteen my menstrual periods started and also an increase in urinary urge and frequency plus abdominal pain was added to my monthly problems. My many trips to my primary care doctor were to check for what appeared to be symptoms of a urinary tract infection. There was abdominal swelling, lower abdominal pain along with pain located in my lower back, and burning when I voided. Often the symptom list included nausea and vomiting, perhaps caused by the severe pain.

In my later teens and as I approached twenty years of age my medical history began to show frequent kidney and bladder infections. These painful times came with the bells and whistles of abdominal swelling, blood in my urine, low back and pelvic pain. At the age of seventeen I was hospitalized for five days due to severe abdominal pain. On the fifth day of my hospitalization I was scheduled to have my appendix removed, because no specific source of the cause of my constant pain was found. On that fifth preoperative day the pelvic pain began to disappear in step-by-step phases, just as it had arrived, and the surgery was cancelled.

At the age of eighteen I was diagnosed with a series of twenty kidney and/or bladder infections in a row. A complete exam of my kidneys proved they were functioning normally. The plan of action was for me to have an ultrasound of my kidneys every six months to try determine why the cycle of infection symptoms continued. As I look back, I do not think that any of my urine specimens were sent out for culture. To the best of my memory they were all tested in the physician's office. This would mean there was no documented verification through the growth of bacteria in a laboratory environment to prove that I did have a urinary bacterial infection.

As often happens with females who have pelvic pain, the focus was on my reproductive system. I do have Polycystic Ovaries (PCOS). What is *Polycystic Ovary Syndrome?* My understanding is that the condition occurs when an imbalance of hormone levels in a female's body causes cysts like balloons to fill with liquid to form in the ovaries. When this was discovered as a reason for my irregular and often painful times of menstruation, I connected all my pelvic problems to PCOS. My bladder being a source of pelvic pain never was considered.

One day in my late teens I ate one of my family's favorite meals, chicken and asparagus baked in a foil packet. I began to sneeze and could not stop. My Mom gave me two capsules of nonprescription Benadryl. Her quick response was because she understood the family history of food sensitivities. That reflexive act saved my life because within five minutes I could hardly breathe. I began to cry and I was so frightened. When the paramedics arrived they said the Benadryl was the key to not having my throat swell shut because of an allergic reaction to what was later discovered to be the asparagus. This frightening event was my introduction to appreciating that what I eat and drink makes a big difference in my life.

My Mom was diagnosed with interstitial cystitis two months after my 911 call and directly I was diagnosed with IC. Her discovery gave an answer to my childhood and teen years of wondering what in the world was wrong with me. For years my symptoms were blindly treated without knowing the reason for the pelvic pain.

The question was asked if there have been any life changes made because of knowing I have IC. The changes in my life because of IC focus on an understanding and an appreciation of how my body reacts to food and stress. I can say I am fortunate because IC really has not stopped me from making any life's choices.

When it comes to the question of how my IC has affected my family I can say that we may have a unique situation because of identifying IC as part of the family genetics. I think that the message that needs to be acknowledged about IC is that many families can have this bladder disorder, as surely as allergic responses can be reflected in family members.

My primary support is my husband. He recognizes that when I have a flare I need extra help. I do appreciate that if your partner does not understand what is going on, the intrapersonal tensions can build. I respect how those closest to us see a change in how we respond to everyday life and wonder what has created such a negative personality. They cannot see pelvic pain, but they do experience its outcomes.

What I have learned to share is a straightforward explanation about the reason for my pelvic pain. I explored with my husband the basics of the known medical thoughts on IC and how it affects me. As an example, the changes in premenstrual hormone levels can often be the tipping point when combinations of stress, yes, even every day get to work on time, dinner on the table, stress, foods we eat, amount of water we drink, and even lifting groceries, can increase pelvic pain or influence a flare. When your partners understand the physical reason for the problem they are more likely to be open and can accept the wave like action if a bladder flare happens. It is a blessing that I have an understanding husband. He is educated about IC.

The knowledge about BPS/IC my Mother has learned is always put to use at family gatherings. Her understanding of IC is reflected in not taking for granted food choices or preparation; by extension this makes every meal a true family affair. My family understands I am as allergic to asparagus and Brussels sprouts as I am to certain antibiotics. This is me and my individual needs. We are all different.

I have listened too many who say that when they should be asleep they find that they feel that they have worked a 24/7 shift because of getting up to void numerous times when they wanted to rest. I have dodged that misery. It is my cats that wake me up. The one upgrade I can recommend is to invest in a pillow top mattress or as we did add more mattress padding. When I have a resting place that cradles my body it helps me relax for a good night's rest.

An ongoing decision is what medications help keep my IC symptoms under control. My list of medications is a short one. Elmiron was one of the first medications prescribed for me. I think it has been the greatest help because over the years it has brought me to a place where I can say I am mainly pain free; with my history this was no small accomplishment. Another of my daily medications is an antihistamine, now sold without a prescription, brand name Zyrtec. Zyrtec's job is to keep my food and seasonal allergies in check and by doing so it appears to help to also keep pelvic pain from flaring up.

On the opposite side, Ditropan was prescribed to reduce my bladder spasms so that the number of trips I made to the bathroom would be less. It didn't work and made me feel as dry as a potato chip. I do not use Ditropan. Elmiron and Zyrtec are my two choices for IC symptom control of pelvic pain, abdominal swelling, and frequently needing to void. My solution to the decision to what meds to take is simple: if it works use it as prescribed. If it doesn't seem do what its job or side effects begin, inform the doctor and tell him what is going on.

When it comes to the anxiety of trying a new medication, my work in the health field helps me understand the why behind trying something new. I make the effort to learn the background of the medications that are prescribed for me and the short and long term effects. My one additional supplement vitamin has both iron and minerals. I have heard that there are some women with IC who cannot tolerate some B vitamins but I have not stirred up any IC problems with my daily prenatal vitamin.

I think that the most important aspect of IC symptom control is my diet. In my life what I eat and drink is the main reason that I can work for long hours as a scrub nurse in an operating room environment and function without problems. I have used the internet and the ICA Network to help me make smarter choices.

Am I a reader of the contents of packaging? Yes indeed. I am very aware of the ingredients that drive my bladder wild; this includes MSG, and preservatives. Do I drink sodas from time to time? Yes. What works for me is if I drink a diet cola, I follow it with bottle of water. Yes, I void more, but it is diluted at that point. Also I give the fact that I take Elmiron is a deciding factor in the ability to wander a bit from the recommended IC list of foods and drinks.

I was no pillar of water drinking virtue but I have increased my fluid intake to an average of six to ten bottles, of sixteen ounces each, of water per day; that amount equals three quarts or more. Sounds like a lot of liquid but Los Angeles is a desert and we live, drive, and work in air conditioning that has dehydration as the major goal to help keep us cool. To this atmosphere of dryness add in the physical demands of my job and hydration is necessary even if IC were only a set of initials.

Water is truly what every cell in our body craves. I have learned it is the simple changes that can make a big difference. When I have gone too far with acid foods, carbonated drinks or chocolate my bladder pain starts within twenty minutes. One element of my personal rescue is to drink water and dilute whatever is causing the bladder discomfort.

I do understand that there is being "overloaded" with drinking water and an electrolyte balance needs to be factored in. That is why, for me, salted almonds or pretzels are a good snack. The two are examples of how to control both stomach acid and to also balance the amount of water with needed salts.

The operating room is my chosen work setting. The work demands are very physical. I am always walking, standing, bending, lifting, and many times running with stress as the nature of the tasks. It is exacting work and I enjoy the challenge. How I deal with a long day can be answered in a bathtub soaking. Water not too hot and a cup or more of baking soda and I can feel the muscle and emotional tension literally drain away.

Because of my medical schooling I have an understanding of human anatomy and physiology. I know why my body responds in negative or positive ways. The point is to take the signals from your body seriously. When you begin to take control, feeling sorry for yourself becomes a sometime thought not a way of life. The more educated you are about our body, the greater appreciation you have for those who love and support you and the special someone you love.

What I Think:

1. Learning stops when the anxiety about the need pee is the only thought.

2. BPS/IC symptoms affect the life of the entire family

3. BPS/IC can be part of our genetic heritage.

4. BPS/IC does not suddenly start at the age of consent, but hormones and my menstrual cycle push my bladder in both positive and negative ways.

5. BPS/IC is part of my body's sensitivity response to food, environment, and tension.

6. Time invested in learning how our bodies work from academic sources and individually helps to make sense of the medical confusion that surrounds pelvic pain.

7. Your water source and amount you drink not only dilutes the urine but when water has minerals or "spring' water it's slightly less acidic. Both elements help the damaged bladder lining to heal and control greater inflammation.

8. Medications prescribed for IC symptoms, and for that matter all conditions need to be understood as to the reason it was prescribed; how it should work and does it interact with any of your other medications?   Follow the prescribed directions and above all don' stop or change a medication before you check with your physician.

9. "We are what we eat." A true statement today as it has always been.

10. BPS/IC needs focused treatment and then you take control.

6. Daniel, age 13
A Child's IC Experience as Told by His Mom

Daniel is now thirteen and my youngest. He is an active and loving adolescent that makes his family proud. I am as protective as mothers are of their children and when there is a health problem, the need to surround them with even more care is in our nature. As an infant Daniel had wet diapers all the time. I remember sitting by the pool with his little bottom exposed to the sun with the hope that his diaper rash would heal. As I remember he seemed to pee every five minutes. When I flash back to that time I now realize that I did not recognize that our son's voiding was troubled. My thoughts were to help his little bottom heal and not the reason for the problem.

At six months old, Daniel had bronchitis. Penicillin was ordered; he had an allergic response that was a total body rash. I still question if that skin reaction was a sign that his almost constant wetting and allergies were connected.

The potty training was very stressful when I realized my child was in pain. Not only couldn't we find a bathroom fast enough, being near a bathroom sent the signal he had to go. There was urge, frequency, and then came what we now know were flares. We learned that a flare for Daniel is bladder pain and spasms that cause him to be unable to void. I have not experienced the misery of retention but I can only imagine the pain of wanting to void and your body fighting the urge.

As a parent of a young child I relied on the pediatrician to guide me. Before Daniel's diagnosis, his pediatrician seemed to hit a wall when it came to identifying the reason for his distressful voiding pattern. After the diagnosis of IC was made I went to her and explained our family connection with IC. Daniel's pediatrician expressed great interest in IC. She said that she had many youngsters in her care that had similar problems with their urinary tract, and they had no bladder infections; she wondered if IC might be the cause. This would seem like a moment when information that would benefit many others would be the result of one youngster diagnosis becoming clear, but it did not work out that way.

The pediatrician researched the topic and stated that the National Institute of Health's (NIH) definition of IC excluded IC unless you were eighteen years of age or older. She reported that clearly the NIH list included a statement that IC occurs in young people after the age of eighteen. In short, Daniel, because of his young age of five, was the not the usual for the diagnosis of IC or perhaps the diagnosis was wrong?

This ended our moment to bring help to the "many" children with voiding problems that she eluded too. I wish at that time that I had been able to challenge her, because I found out years later that the National Institute of Health IC definition list has only one focus, that is to give the standards by which clinical trials can be developed. Yes, IC for those under eighteen must be dismissed, not because a youngster cannot have IC, but because a person must be of the legal age, eighteen or older, to give consent to be involved in a clinical trial. I wonder to this day if the good doctor ever went back to reread that NIH list and realized she had misread the intention of that statement. I also wonder how many other pediatricians have followed the wrong information.

Since his oldest sister and I were diagnosed with IC we recognized Daniel's symptoms; and as they became more intense we knew the next medical stop would be an urologist. I will never forget that at the age of five, after his bladder exam, the hospital dietitian came in with a list of IC forbidden foods and treats. She said, "Well, you can't have chocolate any more." As simple as this statement was, I recognized at the age of five, he had taken in information about IC.

I cannot claim that suddenly my son made a smooth transition by turning to us for diet help and that he embraced a strict IC diet with a smile. When he cried with bladder pain, because he had slipped a flare causing food into his diet, it took many of these painful experiences for the connection between food and bladder pain to be made. After a family party we found him drinking what was left in a bottle of Pepsi Cola. Quickly, that event caused a severe bladder spasm. Our first aid was to have him consume lots of water and a soaking in a bathtub of lukewarm water with baking soda. He has never tried Pepsi again. The adage that nothing teaches like experience is true, but for a youngster, memory is short.

Food plays a major part in controlling the flares of IC for my son. Daniel has learned to side step his flare reaction to spicy and acid foods by his own choices. Somewhere along the line I learned, and think we have all lived the fact, that our taste buds change with what we are exposed to. Our diets in the United States are over salted, over sweetened, over spiced, and over preserved, with chemicals such as citric acid and Monosodium Glutamate (MSG). All of these items may not be totality eliminated from our diets, but our children are healthier for not having been exposed to a constant intake of over seasoned and processed foods.

Is Daniel deprived of fizzy drinks? No, his drinks of choice are root beer, A & W brand, with ice or Sprite. As a food example he also enjoys plain cheese mozzarella pizza, and has had no negative reaction to Oscar Meyer brand hot dogs, on a bun, plain. When he is at a party or Scout camp, he has learned to choose foods that are the least likely to cause bladder problems. I give him credit for knowing he needs to take his own snacks when there might be a question of what food is available.

Daniel has for the past three years been prescribed three IC specific medications: Elmiron, imipramine (Tofranil) and the antihistamine, Zyrtec. Elmiron is thought to cover the thinned bladder lining so that healing is helped. Imipramine is to lessen bladder spasms. Zyrtec is for seasonal allergies and the possibility that histamine release because of allergies also plays a part in the increase in IC symptoms.

Daily life for my child means dealing with school. I have communicated to his schoolteachers at the beginning of every school year the limitations and demands that come with IC. My straightforward discussions have made for greater school contact and fewer hurtful events when voiding is involved. In addition I think these mini-seminars help the adults that surround him at school to be aware of other children with voiding problems in P.E. classes. Because there are others in his classes that also require some extra help, he is not alone.

His friends have known since grade school that he has always had a bathroom pass. Because bedwetting can still be an issue, as precautions if on an overnight in an unfamiliar situation, Good Nights pull-ups and medication help control his bladder spasms give a sense of security.

Amusements parks and outdoor events, on the other hand, are more of a challenge. We have had to leave a waiting line many times to pee before our turn for a ride. This is where a handicap pass helps to make a day planned to be fun, truly a fun day. One solution I have found that helps relieve anxiety is a restroom access card from the Interstitial Cystitis Association (ICA). When attending a parade, for example, we do scope out of where the port-a-potties or bathrooms of choice are located. It is very helpful to know these locations for building a sense of confidence so that we can all enjoy the event. Yes, this does make for a bit more work, but with a little planning the voiding problem is addressed and we move on.

Daniel and his Dad are a team in Scouting and participate in many outdoor activities such as a special overnight and sail on a schooner. They have had many great times, but it is hard on my husband when his son is in pain. For years Daniel would not pee unless he was in stall with a door or a port-a-potty; and never would he go out-of-doors. When he was able to pee against a tree it was a proud day for both of them.

The trust and support between Daniel and his father are built on many years of being together on outings. My husband and I learned long ago that asking for help from the Scout leadership helped smooth the way for both the activity at hand and teaching all of us how to communicate.

One of our main responsibilities as Daniel's parents is continued vigilance for changes in any health issues. The balance when you are a parent of a teenager is to gauge when you step in and take charge or when you guide your youngster to make choices; even when his understanding of the consequences may not be completely appreciated.

The decision making process as parents when health is involved often requires the help of a physician. I encourage building an ongoing relationship with the doctor who is the most knowledgeable about the health history of your child. I appreciate how changes in insurance plans can make this difficult. A great help in the cause of the connecting health, health care events, and medical care is to keep an ongoing record of medical visits, treatments, and medications. A simple folder or binder that stores the records of the health history of your youngsters is a valuable guide for the health care resource and you.

This year was a big transition to junior high school. Daniel has six teachers and has learned he must speak up to clarify any problems that arise. Life has moved on with less bladder pain events, urge, and frequency. Daniel, at thirteen, doesn't realize that he has learned many lessons that come to most of us much later in life. The lessons he is learning are, (1) to a large degree, we are what we eat and drink, (2) listen to you body's messages, and (3) no one can read your mind, you must speak up.

To: _____

Date: _____

Regarding: _____

Bladder Pain Syndrome/Interstitial Cystitis (BPS/IC)

Interstitial Cystitis is a urinary bladder disease of unknown cause characterized by urinary frequency, urgency, pressure and pain in the bladder and pelvic area.

The pelvic pain often increases as the bladder fills and reduces temporarily after voiding. People with IC may also have nocturia or getting up to void when you want to be asleep, pelvic dysfunction, and tension making it difficult begin urination.

This condition causes inflammation of the lining of the bladder and leads to the urinary symptoms.

Common foods that are high in acidic content and can irritate the damaged bladder wall include alcohol, coffee, tea (some herbal teas), all sodas (especially diet), citrus juices (such as orange), tomatoes, chocolate and potassium rich bananas. Also, there certain vitamins such as B & C that can activate the condition, as well as commonly used flavor enhancers and tenderizer, monosodium glutamate (MSG).

Pain medication may be needed to relieve the painful flare of IC.

Individual Adaptation:

1. _____should be allowed to use the restroom as needed.
2. It is recognized that the feeling of urinary urge, frequency and pelvic pain causes distraction and loss of focus.
3. Please allow_____ to have a water bottle in class.
4. If he/she has a bladder flare, please allow him/her to come to the health office.
5. Running, jumping and lifting can also cause bladder pain, increased urgency, and frequency.
6. If his/her pain is severe, please call the parents.

Thank you for your attention to this important matter

_____   _____
Physician   Date

_____   _____
Parent   Date

What I think:

1. Chronic health problems can be evident even in babies. Struggles in attaining the growth and development targets are a signal to investigate the reason for the problem.

2. The identification of a health problem and workable plans of action for a child takes hard work, patience, and creativity.

3. Listen to your child. As an example the line between teasing and bullying can be blurred when dealing with body function issues. Have you helped develop tools to use to deal with questions from others, young and old?

4. A simple filing system for medical records, treatment, blood work, etc. will help your sanity.

5. Family activities need to be realistic when pre-planning. This includes water, food, rescue techniques, and the hours need for travel, etc.

6. How and where a food is grown, processed, packaged, prepared, and the amount consumed all are part of how your child's body reacts to eating or drinking it

7. Take time to listen. Stress is often a trigger for adults with IC. It would be reasonable to know your youngster may face the same feeling of turmoil as he deals with family and school.

8. The appreciation that the standard school environment is for the "well" child. The adjustments needed to produce a safe and instructive school day for your child can be aided with an advocate. In our case it was the school nurse.

9. The school nurse has earned my hero award because of her suggestion of #10.

10. The following is what school nurse wrote as information about IC. Please consider the use of the following from as a guide for young youngster.

7. Laura M., age 67
A BPS/IC Narrative in Two Parts

Background

This is the story of a wife, Mother, grandmother, and businesswoman, who has a tap dancing passion. She relates her frustration with the lack of knowledge and understanding about IC in the medical community, including the specialty of urology. Then Laura took charge.

Laura M.'s Story

My name is Laura and I am 67 years old. I was diagnosed with IC when I was 61 and feel very fortunate that I was an older age when I contracted this disease. Thinking back through my life especially my childhood I cannot recall any particular problems with my bladder. As to allergies, there must have been some slight problem as my mother had me tested when I was around 10 years old. The only things I remember being allergic to chocolate and dust – very common.

My story of IC really begins with my experiences with a specific medical group's health plan that I belonged to seven years ago as I was quickly developing a major problem with frequency. I was sent to one of the urologists in the group and he kept prescribing the antibiotic, Cipro. I remember that antibiotics were prescribed five times within a year, even though I had only had one bladder infection that was officially noted.

Soon the frequency problem escalated to bladder spasms and then to pain – unrelenting pain from the middle of my lower back down through the pelvic area and down thought my thighs. Was this cancer, I kept asking myself? The doctors kept ordering urine tests that showed normal findings.

In my numerous doctor visits, the various medication combinations eventually include ibuprofen for pain, which I was to learn later was disastrous for the bladder. The urologist at the time performed a cystoscopy as an office exam with no anesthesia. I thought I was going to die right there on the table from pain. His opinion after this awful exam experience was he saw nothing unusual.

By the summer of the following year I was in pure misery, and not getting much sleep. My primary care doctor had disappeared and no one knew where he was. I had no primary care doctor. I put in six frantic calls directly to my urologist trying to get an appointment. By this time I was desperate. He did not return any of my calls. Finally his nurse, who was less than polite, told me if I was in that much pain I should see my primary doctor. Pain drove me to seek help and I was left to a medical system that would make a healthy person cry.

I was about to switch to another primary care doctor when they located my original physician in another one of the health plan's facilities. After another night of absolutely no sleep I limped into his office only to be told by him that this was "way beyond his expertise." Now this I believed.

An MRI was ordered and it was normal. I was sent to two gynecologists, and saw six or seven urgent care doctors and emergency room doctors in the 16 months prior to leaving the medical group's health plan. The only advice that I ever received that was helpful was from one of the emergency room nurses who advised me to stop eating anything with acid in it, which I did. This single piece of advice actually gave me moderate relief for a while.

My last visit to my health plan's urgent care facility was several days later. My husband drove me there and I needed a wheelchair because I could not walk. I was bent over with pain and crying, and crying. I begged this emergency room doctor to put me in the hospital; I knew there must be something horribly wrong with me. His response – "I can't do that." I went home with nothing.

I have never been as disgusted with a group of doctors as I was with this medical group. They truly did not know what they were treating. These are samples of the responses I received during my 16 months of physician visits:

- The urologist said, "You have an overactive bladder." This was the end of his discussion and his search.
- The primary care doctor finally admitted, "This is way beyond my expertise." What he was saying was, "I am done."
- The gynecologist took the tact, "You need a behavioral therapist and antidepressant pills." This I thought is very odd since I had never been depressed in my life.
- One of the urgent care doctors stepped forward with the opinion that - "You need a hysterectomy. I am positive. I've seen a thousand women like you. Your scar tissue from your C-section 44 years ago has grown into you uterus."
- Another urgent care doctor simply said, "Bad luck."

- Another gynecologist must have decided silence was golden because he gave no opinion, no advice, and no direction.
- Five more urgent care and three emergency room doctors embraced the no opinions, no advice stance. It was a lonely time.

The kicker to this intense, painful experience was that I told my urologist I thought I had Interstitial Cystitis. In October, My husband and I had been on a Mexican Rivera cruise, the first year of my increased frequency symptoms. While at sea I thought I had a bladder infection and went to see the ship's doctor, who was from South Africa. He told me that it sounded like I had Interstitial Cystitis and to run this thought by my doctor when I returned home. I had never heard of IC, but I looked it up on the internet and it sure sounded like what I was dealing with. I did mention it to my urologist and his response," Only old ladies get that." Imagine! A cruise ship doctor could diagnose me but none of my doctors could. (Or would)

After sixteen months of pain, I had removed myself (and my entire company) from the medical group's insurance and obtained a Preferred Provider Organization (PPO) policy, all within 5 working days. By July 1, I was in my old gynecologist's office, and low and behold, he knew instantly what was wrong with me. His famous words to me – "All" (the other entire medical group) are good for is delivering babies." This doctor sent me to a good urologist – which begins part two of my story.

I started seeing my urologist and my diagnosis of IC was confirmed. His noted quote - "You had IC stamped on your forehead and no one saw it." I wondered if the other physicians were truly blind to my problem or didn't want to see IC.

I was so ill by this time. Sleep? I forgot what it was to have a decent night's sleep. My life was making it to the bathroom as I was "going" between 50 and 70 times in a 24-hour period of time. He immediately put me in a clinical research study. I was never so glad to get to a doctor's office for the twice a week trial visits. The clinical trial used a FDA approved IC medication, Elmiron in an additional way; the medication was instilled directly into my bladder along with taking it orally. This bladder concoction was put in my bladder and helped relieve the pain for a few hours. Along with Elmiron, there were other bladder rescue medications prescribed such as lidocaine. This office staff literally wrapped their arms around me and took care of me, giving me hope and relief.

When I started to really learn about IC, I was determined to give my bladder every break. Knowledge is power as the saying goes. I joined the Interstitial Cystitis Association (ICA) and scoured every edition for anything that would help me. I changed my diet radically and started a food journal that I kept for six months. I grocery shopped at Whole Foods Market that specializes in organic and foods with less additives and preservatives. I read food labels and purchased as much true organically grown food as possible. My food bill doubled but I didn't care. I would rather pay for organic food in my diet than medical office co-pays, more prescription costs, and deal with bladder spasms.

My diet focused on the elimination of preservatives, food coloring, certain spices (spices can be acidic) and any ingredients like soy, or MSG that can be harmful to my injured bladder lining. Condiments were out. For this healing time, multivitamins were out of my daily routine. To this day calcium, vitamin D and E are the list of my supplements.

When it comes to fluids, the Arrowhead Mountain Spring brand of spring water is my choice, Gerber's baby pear juice, peppermint tea, and when I want a cup of coffee, it is Kaffree Roma. In the last several years I have been able to tolerate a little root beer (caffeine free) and Riesling (white) wine.

I carried my list of recommended foods with me and constantly referred to it. When it comes to solid foods, most bread was out; except for sour dough bread from Whole Foods Markets, which has only three ingredients. Fruit was initially eliminated except for pears and honeydew melons. I have added a little banana and apple and some times a bite of peach or strawberry seems to be okay. I eat a lot of vegetables; the ones recommended on the IC diet list to be sure that I am getting enough vitamins. One benefit of my restricted diet was a loss of 12 pounds in a short period of time, which was okay. My pants looked great on me.

This turn around of pain control did not happen quickly. Four months after I was formally diagnosed and treatment was started for IC I was still very ill; in fact I went to the emergency room twice and one office visit because my bladder was in such spasm that it was "locked up" and I could not pee. Sometimes I would be in the bathroom for an hour trying to get one little drop of urine out. I religiously took my

Elmiron and other medications that were prescribed – some of them worked and some did not. Ultrascet generically, Tramadol or Ultram, was a lifesaver for severe pain. Detrol LA was not good for me; it was to relax bladder spasms but it stopped me from peeing. A prescription grade antispasmodic and antiseptic, Pryridum was not good for me. Claritin, an antihistamine, oxazepam for anxiety, amitriptyline or labeled Elavil were all prescribed to help control my runway symptoms. And over the counter antacid, Prelief was and is helpful.

Simple as it sounds baking soda and ice packs really helped. I would take a teaspoon of baking soda and mixed in some water and drink it down. Also soaking in a tub with lukewarm water with liberal amount of baking soda added helped me and was used often. The baking soda neutralized temporality the high acid content of the urine and I think that the relaxation and lower acid water washing over my unhappy pelvis brought some, if temporary, relief. Every night I went to bed with my wonderful frozen gel pack from the IC Clinic – that ice pack was a lifesaver.

With time and my bladder symptoms under control most of the prescribed drugs have been eliminated. I am still on Elmiron twice a day. I always carry my Prelief with me. And baking soda is still occasionally a rescue that really helps.

I want to address a thank you to my husband. He was wonderful throughout this ordeal as were my son, family, and friends. I know my husband felt so helpless; there really wasn't anything he could do. But I got lots of hugs, and kisses and foot rubs and sympathy. He would cry right along with me when I was so miserable. He was so good about the changes in how I cooked for us. When I could, I would cook his food differently than mine, with a bit more spice. As an example, meatloaf was divided down the middle, my side with salt and garlic, which I used plenty of, and his side with peppers onions, ketchup. With his Italian came his tastes for pasta with tomato sauce, and hot spices. My pasta was cooked plain with olive oil and fresh garlic, basil, or rosemary. He didn't mind if I cooked, "plain." He just added more pepper for his individual dish.

It is funny how we crave foods that we never wanted, before simply because we cannot or should not have them. I never particularly cared for chocolate, but after being diagnosed with IC and the food "don't" list included chocolate, how I craved it. I indulge this desire for chocolate with a little white chocolate, which is definably not the same as dark chocolate. Ah, and lemon meringue pie, always my favorite -

off the list. When grocery shopping, I would stand and practically drool looking at a lemon meringue pie. I swear I could have eaten the entire pie standing in the store.

Restaurant dining came back into our lives when I began to have less pelvic pain. For a long time I really couldn't do much of anything, but eventually all that began to change and enjoying a night out returned. There are some rules however: Pain or no pain did I really want those barbequed ribs? The "bland is boring" life style needed to be modified a bit. All I have to do is think of the bladder spasms that would follow, dismissing the no spice rules to keep in check. I usually order plain, not marinated, meats, pasta, baked potatoes, or rice, salad with olive oil on the side, and vegetables. I am sure to have my Prelief with me. Dessert is usually vanilla ice cream or custard pie. I bring my own peppermint tea or Kaffee Roma coffee with me.

Six years and much experimentation have brought me to the point where I have been able to eat at many restaurants that specialize in Mexican, Chinese, and even Thai food. This is such a treat, even being in an ethic restaurant after so many years of shying away from them. I am extremely careful and am not backward about questioning the source and preparation of the food. Often it is a matter of simply having sauce on the side or eating a smaller amount. Well worth these modifications to again enjoy a variety of tastes.

One item I can recommend is writing. It really helped me; in fact I joined a writing class and four more followed. The one-hour respite of my mind being diverted helped to make sense of a chaotic period. We had writing lessons that we had to do at home and it was an activity that engrossed me, and not the pelvic pain that had tried to consume me.

I mentioned in my background about tap dancing. I returned to my dance passion and also exercise as the bladder spasms, pelvic pain, and frequency began to resolve. I have never been one to not have active pursuits and expressing my self with dance was good for my body and soul. It is so good to have it back.

How has my life changed over the last six years? I definitely developed a lot of empathy for anyone that has to live with chronic pain. Before I was always sympathetic, but now I really know how difficult it is to function while living with pain. I am part of a small family business and had to work every day no matter how tired I was or how much pain I was in. When I thought I couldn't make it one more day, I did make it, and I made it the next day, and the next day. Somehow the strength was there to get through and make sense out of my chaotic health. Four years ago my husband became very ill and the next years were really rough. My stress level was high, but I was determined to keep as well as I could in order to help him. He passed away and again I am learning that life takes unexpected new directions.

What I think:

1. Join the Interstitial Cystitis Association (ICA). The ICA offered me informational help at a troubled time from people who understood my dilemma.

2. If your health care source is not responding to your call for help perhaps you need another opinion. For me antibiotics prescriptions clouded the issue of an inflammatory bladder disease that required specific medications and support.

3. Drink lots of good water. By "good" I mean "spring water" The acidity (pH) needs to be close to the neutral that our bladders can tolerate. Stay away from water that is reverse osmosis or labeled "drinking", without minerals it will probably be slightly higher in acid (pH) content.

4. What we eat and drink makes a huge difference in our capacity to heal.

5. At least walk through a store like Whole Foods or Trader Joe's and educate yourself as to organic foods and their costs. Notice how the organic section of your supermarket continues to expand.

6. Keep a food journal. Our support group's website, www.icaction.com, has a 24 hour form that keeps you on track and lists trips to the bathroom and pain level.

7. If you have put aside what you enjoy, plan to return to that activity. As with dance, I returned for short periods of time, stopping if it hurt, and taking the next day off to rest if I needed to.

8. Listen to your body. This might mean an action as simple as an ice pack to your pelvic area.

9. Your family and friend are concerned and more confused than you. Be aware that everyone is doing the best they can.

10. There are days when I wondered what happened to my optimistic attitude. I realized that when I sleep well my outlook returned to a positive nature.

8. Jane, age 47
BPS/IC and Urethral Pain

Background

Jane is a 47 years old, single mother of two sons, 23 and 16 years old. Her active life came to a sudden halt when her urethral and pelvic pain became the center of her daily endurance. Jane has recently returned to school to earn her credentials to work in the health care field. Her story tells how she searched for and created coping and healing skills.

Jane shares how she deals with the nagging urethral pain, options she uses, and her involvement in clinical trials.

At the age of 34, I was a mother of two sons, the eldest with a learning disability, and I was divorced. I had a great job at a prestigious university and loved to be physically active; I was a runner in fact. Then I took a bike ride and my life changed.

Now at 47 I want to share with you my thirteen-year experience of dealing with the pain in my urethra and BPS/IC. My hope is that my story will help give you the strength to move on with your life even when complete pelvic pain control is in the future.

My life turned upside down after a bicycle accident in February 1997. I was showing my older son how to ride a bike. Unfortunately the bike I was about to ride had no seat and my demonstration of how to jump from the height of a curb started a chain of events that brought physical and emotional pain to my future. I fell on the exposed bar and the impact caused bleeding in my vaginal area. All of a sudden I felt a severe throbbing sensation and that feeling has never gone away.

When I was in the in the emergency room I was told that I had torn and severely injured my female area. I learned the specifically injured part of my body was my *urethra*. I learned that the female urethra is a 1 ½ - 2 inches (3-5 cm) tube that connects the urinary bladder to the outside of the body. It is located in women between the clitoris and the vaginal opening. I was told to expect many months of healing.

After the accident I started to have very severe urethral and low pelvic pain when I would empty my bladder; I just figured it would go away in time, but unfortunately it never did. All I had to do was start to pee and the urethral burning would begin. My mind would say just one more drop and the throbbing sensation would be gone. That thought became a wish and that became a prayer; it just didn't happen. The urge was never to leave the toilet.

I must have gone to at least five doctors looking for a reason for my ongoing suffering. They all said there was nothing wrong with me. My urine was not infected and that was the end of the office visits. I thought I was going crazy. There was no light at the end of a tunnel. There were all those physician visits with the message that it was all in my head. It was one of the worst times of my life. I took in well-meaning remarks as, "Well at least you don't have bladder cancer." There was also the friend who said I was lucky to have the throbbing sensation when I tried to explain it using a sexual reference.

I began to search for a reason for my pelvic and clitoral pain and after many frustrating physician visits with no answer I was told I had interstitial cystitis. The procedure that revealed the reason for my mysterious pelvic pain is called a hydro distention. My bladder was filled with water when I was under anesthesia and bladder inflammation was discovered. The inflammation compromises my bladder's protective lining and the nerves are exposed to urine. Interstitial Cystitis (IC) was the label. I now had a diagnosis, but hearing the word *chronic* to describe my pain was the heartbreaking remark that made me breakdown in tears. What I heard was a mouth full of syllables, Interstitial Cystitis, and that there was no cure for this "thing". I remember crying a lot and thinking I am never going to be normal again.

I do believe I have inflammation in my urethra and bladder. I still struggle with the thought that this is my fate for the rest of my life. And I still believe that this entire cascade of pain began when I fell and hit the exposed bar of the bicycle that had no seat. If time could be turned back, I would have never ridden that bike; this is the wisdom that comes at great cost.

I can't tell you the number of times I said the phrase "Why me?" over and over again. There I was with two active children, the little one was five and my older child was thirteen. They were dealing with a Mom who seemed to always be crying because she was in pain. As a parent I have to handle the stresses that come with the individual needs of each of my sons. Seeing their Mom in pain had to be explained. When you have children, crying is not a long-term option.

My son with learning problems could not understand why his Mother was so unhappy. When sharing a health problem with any young child it is hard, they don't understand and ask why you can't get better. I had both situations. I made my explanation as simple as possible by telling both sons that Mommy had a problem when she went to the bathroom; it was not anybody's fault that this happened. I explained how when Mommy pees it hurts and it would go away in time and Mommy would feel better. I also told them that often when I was in the bathroom it took a long time for me to come out and I was safe in that small room.

What I do know is that my urethral burning symptoms can get worse with symptoms of increased stinging and throbbing. I thought these first signs were because of a bladder infection, but when I went to the doctor he would say my urine was fine. I discovered the fact that certain foods and drinks would bother me.

I know I am sensitive to beans, tomatoes, and cheeses. The way these foods bother me is that they literally stop my ability to pee. I decided to write down everything I ate so that I would discover the cause of this shut down of my ability to void.

I found that *any* tomato would cause this peeing struggle. I found that all processed cheeses had some factor that would bring about a problem in voiding. The brand of cheese I have found to have natural ingredients is Tillamook from Tillamook, Oregon and is my safe cheese to enjoy. I do not think I am having a problem with lactose but acids, preservatives, and food dyes obviously have an effect. As an example any kind of beans, other than green, will put my bladder in a state of shock and I can't urinate unless I self-catheterize.

On the positive side, if I stick to simply prepared chicken, turkey, rice, potatoes, saltine crackers, green beans, celery, and steamed spinach and even broccoli my BPS/IC symptoms are less. Sounds plain and it is but it is my safe zone. On the negative side, but oh so tempting, is chocolate – step over the line and I can have the worst IC flare you can imagine.

So the question is: How do I take charge when I cannot pee and/or my pelvic pain is out of control?

1. I fill my bathtub with warm water and a cup or so of baking soda. A 30-minute soak would give me some relief and makes your skin very smooth.

2. A wrapped ice pack on my urethral area, while listening to music can be most helpful to calm down the running wild nerves.

3. Self-catheterizing – I use a onetime use catheter product. It is self-lubricating, a pediatric size, French 6 and the LoFric brand made by Astra Tech. The company has an instructional DVD and even a

magnifying mirror to give you a sense of confidence. I had been married and given birth to two babies and did not have clue what my urethra looked like.

I was taught the technique of putting a sterile catheter into my bladder to remove urine and also to instill medication into the bladder. I was taught the self-catheterizing method to prevent infections at the urologist office and modified it for my needs at home. I have been doing this procedure for the past seven years and often more than one a day.

I have been self-catheterizing for seven years. I estimate six hundred times per year. Why? (1) Rescue (pain reduction) with lidocaine (2) Elmiron and lidocaine mix (3) Removing urine from my bladder for pain control (4) removing urine from my bladder so that not only bladder pain but incontinence is less of an issue.

Writing my story has made me stop and think about my catheterization history. Doing the math, at about six hundred catheterizations a year, times seven years means a total of four thousand two hundred (4,200) catheterizations.

Bladder infections? There have been times that I felt that the urethral burning had increased and had my urine checked and sent to the laboratory for a culture; always it came back no infection. What I was feeling was the added inflammation that comes from the action of putting a tube in to my bladder. I think that one reason for my not having bladder infections is the one use catheter and very small diameter that pediatric size; as small around as spaghetti. Also was told in the urology office about using a mild soap like the Dove or Ivory brand not an antibacterial because of urethral, vaginal and even anal irritation.

4. My method for calming down the bladder pain when I self-catheterize is to mix sterile normal saline with 2% sterile lidocaine in a sterile container then draw it up in a syringe and have it ready to inject through the catheter after I let the urine run out and still have the tube is in my bladder. This makes me feel relief as it numbs the nerves that are the cause if my urethral and bladder pain. This relief can last for at least an hour and often is enough so I can fall asleep.

If you decide on self-catheterization, as a rescue, please remember that one (1) one-half (1½") inches to two (2") is the distance between the outside world and the inside of our bladders. Be patient, be gentle, and be clean. I always have a spare catheter nearby if the first touches an unclean surface.

5. My urologist understands the crazy quilt of symptoms that come with BPS/IC. In about 2001 he opened a research office that tries different avenues of treatment. One treatment that gave me some relief was a mixture of Elmiron (pentosan polysulfate sodium), sterile sodium chloride solution, sterile sodium bicarbonate, and lidocaine put in my bladder with a pediatric, single use non-latex, catheter. The medical term is *Intravesical*. This procedure became the center of a clinical trial that combined oral Elmiron with twice weekly bladder instillations. The focus was to protect the bladder lining so it could heal.

Elmiron, and/or lidocaine bladder instillations offer me some relief. The procedure is simple enough if you are able to safely prepare the solution and able to do a self-catheterization. This insertion of the catheter to drain urine is done for those who do not have the physical ability to void for a variety of reasons to empty their bladders.

I have relied on Elmiron intravesical instillations for the relief of bladder pain for many years. I do self-catheterization at home, camping, or wherever I feel the need to do it. I carry a kit in my car that has sterile lidocaine, sterile saline solution, and sterile baking soda in case my IBPS/IC acts up. I also carry a couple of catheters in case I need to use them. This is my rescue kit.

In recent years I have been a participant in urologic clinical trial that focus on pelvic pain caused by the bladder and urethra. The last trial in which I participated the medication was in pill form; it really helped my IC, but unfortunately it has yet to be approved by the FDA.

The clinical trial I am on now is an injection in the thigh area. This injectable is given to limit growth of pain cells in the bladder and I have three injections to date. The treatment has been giving me some relief as far as not getting up so much during the night to go to the bathroom and the constant stabbing in my urethra has calmed down a little bit, but so far I'm not done with this trial.

Being involved in clinical trials has taught me where those package inserts of lists of side effects come from because after an injection I felt kind of nauseated. I developed numbness in my wrists and reported it to the clinical researcher. After a neurological exam it was diagnosed as having carpel tunnel stress (nerve in my wrists.) My gardening caught up with me and not the medication.

I have to share that during this bumpy time I enrolled in technical school for nursing and after a demanding two years I am moving forward with my nursing degree. My two sons are living at home and we have moved three times in the past five years. I have a great Mom, and we mutually exchange help as we need to. This in three short sentences tells you that life moves on and I am keeping up. There are days that I wonder what my next challenge will be; that is when I take a deep breath and move forward – that is my only choice.

What I think

1. Diet makes a big difference. You can deny it, but take note of your food and drink intake patterns that make for more pelvic pain. I say they are there.
2. As simply as possible explain to your children what is going on. What they don't understand builds scary expectation.
3. Baking soda in a warm bath has healing powers.
4. Consider participating in a clinical trial. The review of your medical history and a good physical can give you information about your health that you never considered and give clues to reducing pain.
5. Long periods of driving or sitting can bring on a bladder flare or aggravate one. The vibration from a car, train, bus and even a plane calls for an ice gel pack, or cold water bottle on my lap.
6. When traveling on a plane, train, bus, arranging for an aisle seating close to the restroom. I have not discovered how to shorten the time I have to sit in a restaurant stall. I am open for all suggestions.
7. Remember the word exercise? For me it is walking and working in my garden I needed to learn that pain means no gain.
8. Before this IC pain hit I was anti medication. Now I know there are medications I require and I make sure I know why I am taking each one.
9. Made a point of educating myself so the word chronic did not mean the scary unknown.
10. A support group helps to reinforce you are not alone. There is hope.

9. Danielle C. age 30
A Never Ending Journey

Background

Danielle is a young woman of thirty who presents herself with a mix of gentle charm and the strength that represents her southern heritage. She connects with so many of us as she works with the complexities of life and reaches specific conclusions about BPs/IC.

Danielle's Story

Hello, my name is Danielle. I have had the blessing of living in the sweet southern green of North Carolina and the fun fast pace of southern California. In my life, I have worked as a tutor, waitress, a glorified administrative assistant for an architectural firm, a closeout and funding specialist, and a beauty consultant. I am blessed with a terrific fiancé and a 13 year-old stepson. I have lived thirty short years, almost twenty of which were plagued with annoying, irritating and the most inconvenient urinary tract infections, or at least that's what I thought.

I begin my story in December 2009 lying in a hospital bed waking up from a diagnostic procedure. Surprised I was not more "out of it," I was able to clearly hear the nurse say, "You have IC." My urologist and his team had already been floating the term around and had given me a ray of hope. But when the words came out of her mouth, it was such a weight lifted off me, a true lifting. It was such a relief to finally know what had been plaguing me for over eighteen years. I really didn't realize what a weight it had been until I felt it lift. When you carry something that long, it just becomes a part of you. It becomes your normal, your everyday. Looking back, it wasn't normal.

I remember getting my first urinary tract infection (at least that is what the doctor told me) when I was in fifth grade. Prior to that, I hadn't really noticed any major problems with my bladder. Occasionally I had to urinate more frequently and sometimes had to lean forward or quickly come back to the bathroom because I hadn't finished. There were comments like "you just went" or "can't you hold it" but nothing major. Then in fifth grade, I was overcome with an incredibly acute sharp pain as I urinated, an unbearable burning followed by a constant and not to be ignored urging to go right back in to the bathroom and try again. My Mother took off work, drove the forty-five minutes to my school to get me, and then the forty-five minutes back to the doctor.

When the doctor finally saw us, I peed into a cup and waited. The doctor came back stating the urine office test (dip test) had come back negative but most likely I had a urinary tract infection (UTI). He sent me on my way with a prescription for the antibiotic, Amoxicillin and a urinary analgesic, Pyridium (phenazopyridine HCL). It appeared to clear up with the medication and the Pyridium stopped the pain. At ten years of age, all I really cared about was getting rid of the pain, not what it was. Sadly, this began a pattern. About every two to three months, my Mom and I would go through the same routine. I have to admit I have an amazing mom who had an understanding boss who allowed her to take off work as much as she had to for this routine. I thank both of them.

Sometimes we had the same doctor and sometimes we got a new one. On one occasion, while still in the fifth grade, one doctor I saw, having heard I was suffering from continuous UTI symptoms, asked if I was sexually active. Can you imagine being ten years old and being asked if you are having sex! In hindsight, although, I'm not sure I would not have asked that question in the same situation with so many UTIs in a young ten year old girl; the doctor was probably as frustrated as my mother and I were in the repetitive way the UTI symptoms kept coming back.

By the time I was in the seventh grade and started menstruating, the visits to the doctor had increased to at least once a month, an occasional emergency room visit because the pain was too unbearable, and numerous visits to a very dedicated nurse practitioner. Minor urinary pain had become a norm but the severe pain had me meeting with my nurse practitioner. She made it her mission to help figure out what was wrong with me. Of all the times I had come to see her, a few samples had come back positive for UTIs but not all of them. It was not a clear-cut case. The battery of tests began. Anything you can think of, I was put through. I even endured a test where they filled your bladder to capacity with warm water. When you were in pain from being too full, they asked you to "pee" on yourself so they would take images of your bladder and urinary tract. Laying there on a cold metal slab naked, "peeing" on myself in front of a staff of four was mortifying enough for a seventh grader but the test left me in pain, too. All the diagnostic tests came back negative, and left Wendy, my mom and me stumped. After everything, I was left with two viable options, a lifetime of daily doses of low grade Amoxicillin or try cranberry pills and lots of water on a daily basis. Not wanting to be on antibiotics the rest of my life, I tried the cranberry pills. For the most part, they seemed to work along with the UTI reducing activities I'd been told to implement. I still had minor pain but after almost three years it had become my normal. I had switched to non-scented regular tampons and cotton panties. The moment I had the urge to urinate, I went. Holding it was not allowed. Needless to say, the trips to the bathroom increased. The major UTIs seemed to have reduced. When I got one, I could "flush" it by bombarding my system with mega doses of water, cranberry pills and Alka-Seltzer. In hindsight, I probably would have been better off without the cranberry pills.

When my mother and I left North Carolina for California, I found myself with a severe UTI. The doctor I saw referred me to an urologist. At the time, I was sixteen and in my junior year in high school. The urologist asked me multiple questions, all the ones that had been asked before. He suggested a battery of tests, all the tests that had been done before. I asked "Why?" He said, "Well, we need to know why you are getting these UTIs." I asked, "Will knowing what causes them change the treatment." His answer was, "No." I thanked him for his time and departed. I couldn't see a benefit to tests without purpose and so I continued my life of minor irritating pain and the occasional severe UTI. During that time, I made many visits to the ER and a few primary care physicians.

The list of antibiotic prescriptions to treat my UTIs evolved over the years. I'd used a series of antibiotics such as Macrobid (Nitrofurantoin), Bactrium (Fulfamethoxazole & trimethoprim); and even Cipro (Ciprofloxin). Pyridium that had been my "go to" rescue for relief of the urgency and frequency symptoms now produced a violent allergic reaction. In my need for pain control, I had moved up the scale of pain suppressants to the opioids, Vicodin (acetaminophen & hydrocodone) or Tylenol (acetaminophen) with codeine. Sadly, and in my ignorance, I'd go to the ER, tell them I had a UTI, and what had worked in the past to relief my symptoms. I would give a urine sample and, positive or not, they would send me home with my usual cocktail. The same mantra of words "gives it a few days" and sure enough my pelvic pain symptoms would clear up. Vicodin or Tylenol with Codeine would help enough with the pain that I could function. So life continued. No one ever once mentioned Interstitial Cystitis.

At the age of 20, I developed another troublesome health problem. This time I found that all I could eat was potatoes and chicken broth. Everything else came up. I was losing weight I was not intending to lose and rapidly - about a pound a day. I was generally nauseous and found that my digestive system was pretty much messed up. Nothing worked like it was supposed to and nothing was consistent in its reactions. I went to my new general practice doctor and without examining me, hearing my history or questioning me, she walked in and having read the intake sheet stated, "You are suffering from stress. There is nothing really wrong with you. It's all in your head." I left in tears still no better than before. Through a turn of fate, I found myself at another general practitioner's office, who reassured me that an answer could be found and contact was made with a gastroenterologist, for what would come to be diagnosed as my unknown gastric condition. At the same time, the primary physician, based on my history of UTIs, gave me a standing prescription for Cipro and Tylenol with Codeine so I would not find myself suffering from a UTI on the weekend.

Through a myriad of failed prescription cocktails and painkillers designed to control the symptoms and help me with a normal life, I finally found a technique that worked for me. It consisted of an almost vegetarian, bland, whole gran, virtually gluten free diet, and a series of herbal supplements. My gastric condition got pretty much under control. I felt like I had a great gastroenterologist who looked at all aspects of my life. He did know about my chronic UTIs; but there was never a connection between my UTIs and the gastric condition and the two were still being treated independently of each other. At the same time, I also started developing allergy-induced asthma. I had always had an allergy (interestingly enough to bell peppers) but not to the point I was now experiencing. Again, another specialist (allergist) and again, this physician knew about both chronic conditions and I was given another battery of pharmaceuticals cocktails. Yet no connection was made between my chronic conditions and my new allergies and so they continued to be treated separately from each other.

Ironically, as I ate my very bland and organic diet combined with the herbal supplements I was taking, I didn't have the frequency of severe UTIs as I once did. I still had them but not the frequent severe ones of my past. My water intake had increased and become my only beverage. The acidic foods I previously ate were all but eliminated from my diet and almost everything was organic. Looking back I can remember and pinpoint experiences and feelings of UTIs related to intercourse and menstruation or moments of intense prolonged stress.

I was ignorant and just figured this was a part of life. In fact, in talking with my Mother, aunt, cousin, and grandmother, I discovered that frequent UTIs were common in our family and especially with intercourse and menstruation. We all just figured it was normal. So I continued to live my life with all my health challenges trying to focus on the positive in my life. Then I found my life changing drastically.

Almost eighteen years after my first UTI like episode, I found myself in a loving but extremely stressful relationship, having been laid off from my 8-5 job, my gastric and allergy conditions flaring like never before, back and body aches, and fairly persistent UTI like symptoms. Emotionally, I was operating in a state of functional, verging on nonfunctional, depression. My diet of before had transformed into late night meals of fast food and meats and fats. My personal home-based Mary Kay business began to suffer, I couldn't book appointments when I was in pain and was scared about being able to hold appointments. I couldn't hold appointments when I was worried that I'd have a UTI or gastric flare up that I couldn't control. In fact, I had to cancel an appointment ten minutes before because I had taken a Vicodin for the pain of a UTI that just came on and began horribly vomiting. Needless to say, this added to my stress, which became a compounding issue.

A few years ago, after having intercourse I found myself sitting on the toilet in intense pain. It was like a UTI I had never experienced. The pelvic spasm was so bad; I was in tears and hunched over from the pain. I was bleeding in the little urine I was voiding. I'd washed warm water over my vaginal area, which was throbbing, in equal pain as the burning sensation that erupted from my urethra and radiating over my whole body. Probably from all the straining, my back felt like knives were sticking out of it. I literally and physically could not get off the toilet. By the time I got the ER, I got a stronger version of Tylenol with Codeine, a prescription for Macrobid and orders to go in to see my regular doctor. The next day, I was still in pain though not as severe and sitting at my doctor's when I was notified there was no infection showing. The next words out of my doctor's mouth sent me reeling with emotions. "You know, it might be Herpes" and she gave me a prescription for Valtrex. Imagine, if you will, having to tell your fairly new significant other that you might have herpes, and what's worse, having to tell him that the only way you could have gotten it was from him. Can you imagine the emotions that were going through me? My life was anger, fear, more anger, frustration, dispiritedness, some more anger, and lots and lots of tears. Neither of us could imagine how we got it as both of us had very little experience sexually, knew our previous partners extremely well and I had been tested before.

A week later, I found myself in the physician's office again, the Valtrex having not worked and back in intense pain. This time, she had a different thought. Clearly the herpes had been wrong. I had been in several times over the last five months with UTI symptoms and only one positive UTI. She suggested something called "IC" and that I should see an urologist. Despite my previous experience with urologists and testing for "my condition", and with her reassurance that there were new developments. I had hope for the first time in eighteen years and the possibility that I could have a fairly normal life. The doctor said, "We'll have to have the testing done, but I think your urologist will agree, it's extremely likely and plausible that you are someone who suffers from Interstitial Cystitis."

I went home for the first time excited after a doctor's appointments. Armed with the reading material, I began to read and share with my family. After eighteen years of frustration and many, many, many doctor appointments, I think my mother was more excited than I was. I began to implement the ideas from IC clinic. Though I would not wish it on anyone else, I was relieved to know I was not alone in the world, that others, too, had similar experiences. I began to reflect on my life over the last eighteen years. What had seemed like simple isolated urinary tract infections now had connections that no health care professional or I had ever made. I now understood why I was getting up so often at night and made trips to the bathroom. There was reason behind the allergies and gastric condition and that there was a connection between them. There was a greater understanding of why intercourse could be painful both during and after; why around my menstrual period, or times of stress, that I would have stronger and more persistent flares. I could pinpoint when I did not have enough water for a consistent period of time or overdosed on diet soda that I had been far more likely to experience a flare than not; even why when I was following my bland, macrobiotic diet that my symptoms and flares were reduced.

With the official diagnosis came more options and more education and yes, true hope. Hope that I could live a normal- drink beer, eat pizza, and have a sex-life. I began experimenting, educating myself and my family and friends. I continue to evaluate what I eat and drink. I already drank a lot of water and for reasons of taste I prefer

Arrowhead Mountain Spring Water. Since the diagnosis, I have become far more conscious of just how much I am drinking, and definitely when I'm not getting enough. From the various resources, I have also found out that this choice of taste actually provides my body with minerals and lowers the acidity of water. I haven't given up soda quite yet but I am very conscious about how much I drink and when to stop before I have an issue with respect to my IC. I am aware the caffeine in the sodas can dehydrate my system. Interestingly, I find that when I drink dark sodas versus light colored soda (diet or not) I have a harder time with dark than with light. I know there is generally about double the amount of aspartame, (a sweeter that is in so many products like Equal) in dark diet sodas versus light. Additionally, I can generally handle non-diet sodas better than diet. I assume the sugar is better than the artificial sweetener found in diet drinks. I've also noticed when I drink too much soda I can counter the negative bladder effects with drinking lots of water. As of yet, the levels of potassium do not seem to noticeably affect me. One thing that can truly trigger an IC flare is wine. Anything more than half a glass and I can expect some reaction. Generally, the dryer the wine the worse the reaction and though I prefer whites, reds do not have as harsh a reaction for me. The short version is the more water (spring) I drink, the better I feel.

Acidity seems to be a key component to what I can eat and drink. There were some foods that were easy to determine; the "don't eat under any circumstance" for me is pineapple. If I eat even the smallest amount of pineapple, fresh, processed, or grilled, it leads to a bladder flare. Other diet choices were not so easy to figure out, and truly I still am working on my diet list. The basic food list and food diary from the IC clinic and information shared at support meetings became really important; but all the diet information was a guide to my individual list that I continue to modify and could carry in my phone so I could enter things as they occurred. From my diary, I learned I could have cooked sweet onions or green onions but nothing raw. I had thought I pretty much was going to have to give up tomatoes but after an IC Support Group and the sharing by one member, I was able to add back vine grown tomatoes and grape tomatoes, occasionally cooked as in spaghetti sauce or grilled/baked tomatoes.

Between the medications and environment of Southern California (as opposed to the humid moisture-rich atmosphere of North Carolina), I tend to run on the dry side. Additionally, my body tends to thrive on veggies, fruits, potatoes and whole grains with limited proteins, preferably plant proteins. When I shop I opt to buy fresh vegetables and fruits versus processed foods. Processed foods tend to be high in sodium and preservatives, which dehydrate the body. Fresh produce, raw or cooked without salt, helps provide higher moisture content to the body. I am fortunate that where I live (Southern California) there are lots of options available for the discerning shopper. Stores like Whole Foods, Trader Joe's, and Fresh and Easy provide a variety of options for people who need unrefined grains or organic produce. Plus, I have been pleased with the organic options that groceries stores like Albertsons, Ralphs, and Vons are offering in produce and other products.

Asking what is in something before eating it has been a part of my life for a long time, as I always had to ask about bell peppers. I now ask if things can be modified to accommodate allergies and I have begun to patron businesses that do so more freely. Disneyland and IHOP both are phenomenal when it comes to this. IHOP asks you if there are any food allergies they should be aware of and Disneyland will happily modify food specifically to your allergies if you ask. Disneyland even has a book of every meal cooked in the parks that tells you exactly what the included ingredients are. When I am somewhere that limits what I can eat or it is something I truly want enjoy, say Thanksgiving dinner or at an amusement park like Sea World, Prelief has become a lifesaver. I'm still cautious of what I eat, but I have more flexibility in my choices.

I still struggle with food because I love to eat. I grew up in a family that loved to eat and loved to eat all kinds of food. It's challenging to say no to something you have enjoyed your whole life. With all of my health conditions, my mother has been extremely understanding and lenient in my dietary needs. We've worked together to make the modifications to our family eating to keep me in the most comfort. It wasn't until I started dating that food became more of an issue and this remains one of the greater challenges I face. As I mentioned earlier, I have a very supportive fiancé and stepson, but food is one of the areas where communication seems to breakdown. Both would be happier with pizza, spaghetti, tacos of meat, cheese and hot sauce, cheeseburgers, etc. coupled with lots of eating out. Vegetables and whole grains, healthy meats and proteins are almost non-existent in his household, which makes cooking and eating my IC diet, challenging to say the least. Food is already a challenge and it doesn't give my willpower much of a fighting chance. When I'm still learning about what will affect my body, it's hard to explain I'd prefer not to go out and have him understand. One of the approaches I'm taking is to cook more. When I do the cooking I have control over what's made and exactly how it's made. The best thing, is both he and my stepson are being exposed to healthier foods, eating better, enjoying it and I get the benefit of knowing I'm doing better by my health conditions. When we do eat out, I try to opt for romaine lettuce salads, heavy on the vegetable sides or foods that I have already determined are safe to eat. And as I mentioned earlier, I am not afraid to ask what's in something or if they can modify it for me. Again, Prelief is a great companion.

Food isn't the only thing affected by my IC diagnosis. Relationships and how I communicate have had to adjust. The biggest change in communication had to take place in me. I tend to carry things close to my vest and not share with people what I am experiencing. As a coping mechanism, I grin and bear the mild to moderate pain and irritations about my health. It was not until it got really bad that people truly knew something was wrong. I'd learn to do that in order to function in school, in jobs, and in social settings. Unfortunately, I carried that same trait into my personal relationships. My significant other often said, "Please let me know what's going on?" but I'd keep it close to my chest. I can't fault him for thinking something was wrong when the normal happy, full of life girl became the quiet, non-talkative girl beside him. He really didn't understand what was going on inside of me or why there had been a transformation. I couldn't blame him for getting frustrated when I snapped or didn't want to talk or do things. Nor could I get too annoyed at him when my health made us late or put me in a position where I said we have to leave or couldn't go because I was not in a physical position to be around people. I couldn't blame him for getting frustrated when he wanted to be amorous and I wanted to but felt I couldn't, and acted like I wasn't interested. I chose not to tell him, "It would hurt". I felt, mistakenly, that it hurting was worse than the occasional "I'm tired." I say I couldn't get mad at him but I'm human. Whether he knew what was wrong or why I was requesting it, he should have just said ok and do what I needed, right? Well, no.

As I learned to communicate with him, he surprisingly got more understanding. Novel concept, huh? He's human and has his moments, but for the most part he understands. If I'm having a hard morning, which often is the worst for me, we have learned to adjust our morning to later activities and accepted that sometimes we are going to be late. I know it's difficult for him, and me for that matter, but we are learning to go with the flow. I'm recognizing that telling my significant other that "Today is a challenging IC day." Doesn't make me weak, but helps him to help me. He is willing to help with rescue techniques and relax techniques. When I am having a bad day, he has often, gotten "the kit" ready- heating pad up full blast on the bed, pillows for my legs, ice pack wrapped in towel, and rubs my feet and legs as I try to relax. When it's really bad, he just holds me and lets me cry something very difficult for him since he hates seeing me cry. Intimacy has gotten better as well. While I still have occasions where a flare prevents intercourse, we have learned to enjoy other forms of physical intimacy and pleasure. In fact, sometimes it can be more intimate and close than the actual act of intercourse. We have also learned to be more communicative in what feels good or not for both partners. Interestingly enough, our physical relationship, though good before, has become more varied and "spicy" as a result of accommodating my IC.

Along the same lines, I've had to learn to communicate with my body a lot more and truly listen to what it is saying. If you have never tried this, may I suggest you do. I think you will find the conversation highly enlightening. Previously, I would push myself, often ignoring the signs of my body, and would find myself down and out for the count. After a year of frustration with my health and getting the IC diagnosis, I recognized that listening to my body AND addressing what it said, was critical. Though I am not as diligent as I should be and can easily lapse into my previous poor habits, I have found that relaxing activities are extremely valuable. I have found the benefit of a bi-weekly half hour massage, practicing yoga stretching (especially Namaste yoga as it focuses on breathing, gently moving into poses and is done to calming music) and taking one hour (half-hour minimum) for myself to center. Warm baths surrounded by calming scented candles (ones that I am not sensitive to) are an awesome way to get myself to sit still and relax. The warmth of the water actually forces the muscles to relax while the scented candles help pull my mind away from the day. Often, I will add baking soda to the bath water as a way to combating the acidity in my body. Just as important as pampering your body and relaxing, is taking cues from your body when it gives it. Though it may interrupt my day, if my body is giving me signs that I need to rest and take a break, I have learned the sacrifice of the small break is far less costly than the hours or even days of a severe flare.

Equally important to relaxation is the value of sleep. At its worse, I would get up three and four times a night to pee. Worse to me was the effect of the lack of sleep on me during waking hours. I was exhausted and lacked the energy needed to do even the most rudimentary tasks in an appropriate amount of time - mostly due to a lack of ability to focus. I'd find myself tossing and turning for a comfortable position that would let me sleep. If that went on long enough and I couldn't quickly go back to sleep, the urgency to go to the bathroom would get me up making it that much harder to sleep. Until I had the diagnosis, I had no idea or even suspected that something not working in my bladder could cause pain in my lower back, vagina area, thighs and legs. Besides the relaxation techniques and comforting from my significant other, pillows have become my friends. By placing them in certain ways, I can adjust my body to a comfortable position, allowing me to sleep most of the night. The best position I have found is a pillow under my stomach and sleeping on my stomach. Most of us have been taught that getting a good night's sleep does help reduce one's stress, one of my major culprits in an IC flare. Stress does different things to everyone's body in its effects. For me, stress has always taken its toll on my body from weight gain, to moderate acne, to vomiting and nausea and, in hindsight, persistent Interstitial Cystitis flares. I suspect it increases the acidic side of my pH body level. Managing it is critical for my staying neutral.

One way that has proven absolutely valuable to managing both my stress and my IC has been being prepared. In my case, I have rescue kits -- one at my house, my fiancé's and two travel kits. All of these kits allow me to be prepared at the first signs of flares and not to have to worry "Have I forgotten anything?" My rescue kits at home and my fiancé's place consist of a heating pad, the gel ice pack that was given to me at my first clinic appointment (the best thing I have ever received from a doctor), Tylenol (acetaminophen), Urelle the substitute for Pyridium, my gastric herbal supplements, allergy medication (currently Allegra (fexofenadine-pseudoephedrine) and Flonase (flunicasone)), an over the counter nasal spray, a rescue inhaler, baking soda, and an empty water bottle or glass for baking soda washes. My car always carries a large bottle of water and has a back support and heating and massaging pad for the car. When I travel on extended trips,

I have a similar kit. However, it was on a trip that I discovered my most valuable lesson in fighting and living with Interstitial Cystitis.

The lesson was that of focusing on the positive and making a decision to do so and then manage that decision daily. The idea of positive thinking is nothing new to me. I am an Independent Sales Director with Mary Kay (a skin care and cosmetic beauty direct sales business) and have been an independent contractor with them for eleven years. From my first training session, retraining your brain, thinking and speaking more positively was one of the most highly suggested activities for your success. I have seen the benefit of it in my own personal life and business. I truly try to do that with every aspect of my life and while I am definitely still a work in progress, I have made great strides. About two days before I was to leave to attend our annual Sales Director Training in Houston, I began to experience the beginnings of what at first I thought was a flare. I attempted all my rescue techniques to no avail. As it continued into the next day, I assumed it must be a true urinary tract infection. Since I was going out of town, I arranged to come into the doctor's office for a urine test. I figured that worse case, they would call in a prescription to a local pharmacy in Houston. Needless to say, I was greatly dismayed when the nurse said, "Your urine is perfectly clean. You don't have a UTI." My mouth said, "Oh. Okay." But my brain was saying, "Oh my God. Now what am I supposed to do?" I'd tried all my rescue techniques and I didn't thinking sitting in an arena with over 10,000 women with an ice pack nested between my legs was going to be the most lady-like. And there was NO WAY I was going to miss this event. Clearly, I was not in the best mindset at the time.

So I boarded the plane to Houston after two trips to the bathroom at the airport. I made another bathroom trip on each plane and two more waiting at the airport for my lay-over. I found "comfy" chairs and wrapped a blanket behind my back. I downed lots of water and took my Urelle like clockwork. By the time I was at my hotel, I was in complete agony. And, yes, as soon as I got into my room I made another trip to the bathroom. The truly challenging part of the trip was half way through my first flight, I realized I'd left my Tylenol, my Flonase, my heating pad, my ice pack and most importantly my baking soda. In my hurry to get packed and to the airport, I forgot my travel kit. Ugh. Thank God the pillow was thick and the bed comfy. Between it and the Urelle, I was able to sleep. My roomies, who were three of the best Mary Kay Sales Directors, began to enwrap me in the positive pink bubble that is our world.

The next day I bought Tylenol, took my Urelle and headed to breakfast -- about two hours later than I had planned. Thanks to a wonderful client focused manager of the Hilton Hotel and the training from my Mary Kay business (find a way or make a way training),I was able to procure a very vital form of contraband -- a cup of baking soda from their bakery. I made it through the day and slept surprising well despite the pain. I repeated my Urelle and long trip to the bathroom routine the following morning and further immersed myself into the incredibly positive, upbeat and uplifting environment of my Mary Kay Seminar. By lunchtime, I was inundated with positive people around me in that environment. I wasn't focusing on my pain. In fact, I didn't know it was there, so much so that I forgot to take my follow up doses of Urelle. By the evening, it had dawned on me that I didn't have my flare anymore. It was at that point I made the decision to not only live to personally work on constantly looking at and remaining positive but to also to work on surrounding myself with positive people and environments. It's not that I believe the positive environment fixed my flare. Rather, it's being in the positive environment that allowed me to focus on other aspects of my life, to relax and release stress versus holding it in and adding the negative energy of a negative environment. That's also not to say that I don't have flares anymore, but my focusing on the positive and keep myself in a positive environment helps me move through them quicker.

The journey of my Interstitial Cystitis has been and remains a never-ending journey. I am constantly learning from my body, from support groups and materials, and from other living with the illness. There is no anger toward the doctors who treated me previously as I was very lucky to have, for the most part, doctors that admitted their limitations in knowledge of the body and its illnesses. Though I would have appreciated more doctors who were informed of interdisciplinary advances and discoveries, it is a rare doctor that looks beyond their discipline and treats the body as working with the patient and healthcare with a more holistic approach. Attached is my list of what I think about my IC journey. I hope it gives you the courage to know that the more you learn the journey becomes easier.

What I Think:

1. Don't give up on finding answers to your symptoms. If something doesn't feel like it's working, record what it is doing and how you feel, and share that with your doctor. They don't know everything and each BPS/IC patient is different. Therefore each patient's cocktail of drugs and treatments is different. For me, I have gone through several allergy drugs (allergies seems to be a trigger for a lot of my health problems) currently using Allegra and Flonase coupled with Prelief, and an over-the-counter nasal spray. I highly recommend Elmiron (out of the capsule - gelatin capsule brought on intestinal problems) for anyone suffering from IC who can afford the medication.

2. Put yourself first. Take time to relax and pamper yourself. Get rid of stress as much as possible and inundate yourself with positive self-talk and surroundings.

3. Listen to your body and your gut. If something doesn't feel right, it's probably not. By recording these feelings and "symptoms" of your body, you will learn your warning signs.

4. Educate yourself. Being informed is your best weapon in your fight for a normal life. IC support groups, clinics and the Interstitial Cystitis Association (ICA) are great resources.

5. Don't let anyone tell you it's in your head. Learn to ask for help and to say no.

6. Ask and find a doctor who is familiar with Interstitial Cystitis.

7. Just because you don't have pain in your bladder doesn't mean that it's not your bladder causing it. My back, legs, buttocks, and vaginal area hurt and definitely my urethra area but never really my pelvic or bladder area. Be willing to look and explore outside of just the obvious.

8. If intercourse is painful, something is definitely not right; that's not normal. As you heal be open to other sexual pleasures that do not cause pain.

9. Having had many misdiagnosed urinary tract infections, insist on a culture. IC and UTIs have different treatments and need to be handled differently.

10. Lastly, just because you have lived with something for a long time and you have a family history of similar challenges, doesn't mean it's normal.

10. Grace, age 50
Cancer and BPS/IC: Life Means a New Day

Background

Grace's story begins with the discovery of her road to recovery from BPS/IC; then five years ago her health focus took an unexpected turn because of a colon cancer diagnosis and her story expanded to how to protect her bladder from the negative effects of chemotherapy and radiation treatments. She explains her history of IC and her concerns about how her bladder and gastrointestinal system would react as she continued to work on returning to health through multiple cancer battles.

Graces' Story

At the age of fifty I had to take a disability retirement and say goodbye to the more than twenty five years of working in Special Education. I have had the pleasure of guiding children and young adults who daily take up the challenge of disabilities that include Autism, Cerebral Palsy, being unable to hear or see, and Downs Syndrome. Many of these young people must deal with maneuvering wheelchairs and other physical disabilities. These youngsters taught me the many blessing of life.

In recent years my IC symptoms were under control and then came the diagnosis of colon cancer, colon surgery, radiation, and chemotherapy. My story reports my past and present IC history; the return of the cancer as it took up residence in my pubic bone and then my lungs. I continue to live the philosophy of one day at a time, and I have had to remember that each day is made up of seconds and minutes and then we have a new day.

Before my work became school based, I had to travel multiple freeway miles. Bathroom stops were rare. The urinary urge and what is called frequency was not even in my thoughts. But when I did arrive at my destination I went straight to the bathroom, and that would be the end of my voiding story for long periods of time. I had never heard the term of Interstitial Cystitis (IC) or pelvic pain. How our lives can change...

My IC history seems to be blended with gynecology problems. When I was twenty-seven years old, after multiple episodes of cramping and bleeding, I had a cyst removed from an ovary. After surgery, my menstrual periods were back on schedule and I had no more cramping. Ten years passed and I had a cyst removed from an ovary. Shortly thereafter I had a larger ovarian cyst and there was the addition of anemia because of blood loss from nonstop periods. Because of the low iron I was tired all the time. The solution was again surgery and another cyst removal. My reproductive system should have stabilized. It was not to be, as IC and endometriosis seem to have linked up in a synchronized way to produce double pelvic pain.

The first thought that my bladder was not in the same healthy state as the rest of me was from a gynecologist appointment to confirm whether I had either a urinary tract infection (UTI) or a vaginal yeast infection. I could not really tell how to describe my discomfort. My sample of urine was found to have a small amount of blood and I was given antibiotics. My physician was retiring I was to exchange a male for a female gynecologist. As I remember that office visit I had no urgency or pelvic pain. So maybe it was a bladder infection. No urine culture was sent to the lab, so I will never know, yet I wonder, if this was the first sign of bladder or urethral inflammation.

I do remember all too well, June of that year, while working summer school, I had pain like I had never felt before in my lower pelvic area. The pain took me down to my knees. I was so afraid to move because of the fear of fainting in front of my class. This attack of pain happened on an outing and the kids kept asking if I was OK. I thought that it all must tie in with a bladder infection again and perhaps endometriosis.

In late August my new gynecologist wanted me to have a hysterectomy because the heavy bleeding and severe cramping that was part of my endometriosis continued. At this point I really did not care what she did. I just wanted the pelvic pain and heavy bleeding to stop. At the age of 42, I had a total hysterectomy with the added information that I had pre-cancerous cells on my cervix that were removed at the time of surgery.

Again, I thought this surgery was the close of a painful and exhausting chapter in my life. I seemed to heal quickly from the procedure. I can remember feeling great and full of energy and no pain at all. That "great" feeling lasted for four weeks.

The pelvic pain came back like a lighting strike. If there is any one out there who can relate to the lower portion of your pelvis sending your brain the message that you have a third degree burn in your bladder, you understand. All I could do was curl up in a fetal position on my bed and cry. I called out to my mother to help me.

I remember calling the doctor's office and nurse heard the desperation in my voice. She knew I was in big trouble and the doctor said come right in. I was so cold and shivering because of the pain. They gave me a pain medication to rescue me from my misery.

The doctor reconfirmed that post surgically I was healing well. She said that a urine test was the next item to check to see if I had a urinary tract infection. The on site urine test showed once again a trace of blood in my urine. I commented that in the past when blood was found in urine, as part of my routine office check, my former gynecologist ordered antibiotics; her response was "not this time." The pain medication was helping; even so the doctor said, "See you in the morning."

That night I counted my bathroom visits; the total was sixty-three trips. How after surgery could I still be in pain and be going to the bathroom more than I ever had? I would try to lie down and it was useless. I realized this was going to be one of the most miserable and sleepless nights of my life.

Morning brought a troubling conversation with my gynecologist as she told me that she had spoken with another doctor and they jointly thought that I had Interstitial Cystitis. The next step would be having my bladder examined; that would mean another hospital, another physician, and a cystoscopy exam was in my future.

First I will share that I did not want to have any exam done. I thought I knew my body better than any physician. I went through with my exam and awakened in the recovery room insisting that the nurse give me my clothes so I could leave. I was not going to stay in the hospital any longer. I was so angry about my diagnosis and I verbally snapped at the nurse. I put on my clothes and walked out.

I will never forget that day. I was not going to have a disease label that took away my joy of eating. With IC, the pronouncement was that my food choices ran from limited to greatly limited. I love to explore all types of different food. Dining was a key source of pleasure and a way to enjoy my friendships. I have a good friend and we considered ourselves "connoisseurs" of the foods of the world.

This was a major change in my life and I perceived it as an attack. I come from a Hispanic legacy of spices and plenty of it. Interstitial Cystitis would mean I would miss my way of cooking, dining, friendships, and my very heritage. The word bland did not fit in my life style at all.

After the cystoscopy exam my bladder reacted, as has been reported in medical literature, with the miracle of significantly less pain, urge, and frequency. I knew the urologist was wrong. I continued to eat what I wanted to eat. Then slowly over the months I began to pay the consequences for my vacation with IC symptoms, but not as it turns out from IC.

I reacted to the return of my painful bladder by isolating myself from my friends because reality began to filter in that I did have IC. I was sad that there would be no more Friday "girls' night out" to dine at different restaurants. I gave it a good try to hide my pelvic pain, but the point was I could no longer deny I had pain because of my bladder.

The post cystoscopy appointment to the urologist that I did not want to make, I had to make. I no longer had much of a life. My bladder hurt if I was standing, sitting, or bending. There was no pain free zone. It seemed I could not stop urinating both day and night. There was little to no sound sleep. It seemed that every time I ate, my bladder pain became stronger. I made it to work but little more.

The urologist has an IC Clinic on Tuesday mornings. At my first visit, I arrived on time and my exam room experience began directly. Before I knew it there seemed to be any army of people in that small room. I could not think. I was overwhelmed. I remember my history being taken by two of the patient advocates and a folder being pressed into my hand with the direction that I might want to read the contents. I clearly remember the directive to follow a bland diet for ten days, and keep a food log of everything I would eat, and drink. It truly was too much information.

I finally saw the urologist. His first words were, "Now lady, it (IC) will get better slowly-"I did not hear the word "better"; I heard the word "slowly". One of my medications was to coat the inside of my bladder, which was Elmiron. Atarax (hydroxyzine), an antihistamine for environmental or food sensitivities that can reflect in an increased pelvic pain reaction, and Valium (diazepam.) Both were both taken two hours before bedtime so that bladder spasms could be quieted, I could get some sleep.

This time, I shelved my denial and began to appreciate that unlike endometriosis or cysts, I had a choice of taking an active part in my recovery and stabilizing my bladder. I could now reject having to continue down this painful road. This is when I look in the mirror and said get a grip. I did not know where I was going but I needed to move forward. Little did I expect that change in my behavior toward IC of listening, learning, and taking action would serve me well over these past years.

As a part of the urology office support, there is the Citrus Valley IC Support Group. As part of learning about IC I went to my first meeting and found that the Group's emphasis was an education, such as what the physician sees through the cystoscope, medication choices, and the "why" behind the medications prescribed. This is what I needed to give me a base of understanding.

I was able to say out loud to the group the symptom that I thought was so strange, that even the medical professionals would dismiss it. Part of my painful bladder symptoms was a vibrating pelvic sensation. At several meetings was a man in attendance, though there were more women. I was surprised that men have IC too. He spoke up and described that his pelvic pain felt like putting his hand on a wall that had a motor running next to it. He explained it caused stress and distress because it was a constant interruption to sleep. I had a symptom match and validation. I found that inflammation and nerves are linked; the first of many of my "ah-ha" moments.

As I worked my way back to a civilized bladder and my life, I had to confess that I was a constant cigarette smoker. The only time I remember Jo, from the urology office, being beyond annoyed with me is when I admitted my smoking as I declared my misery with a flare of bladder pain. She said she was throwing empathy and sympathy out the window unless I stopped. There was only so much education, medication, and support could do. It was again up to me.

I give great credit for my bladder healing and decrease in bladder pain to diet changes and medication; slowly I did improve. I found that my taste buds began to appreciate the subtlety of herbs such as basil, thyme, with garlic for a subtle kick instead of jalapeno peppers, curry, and ginger. I was becoming more sophisticated in my food choices.

I did not stop cigarette smoking until the day of my colon cancer surgery. I left my hospital room, went outside and had my last cigarette.

My IC history was initially a large part of my concern as chemotherapy and radiation was scheduled after colon surgery as part of the treatment plan. The thought was to protect my bladder lining from the both the chemicals and radiation that scatters even with the more precise application now available.

There were two parts to my bladder protection plan; Elmiron was key for me. My prescription for BPS/IC was four Elmiron capsules every day; two in the morning and two in the evening. The urologist recognized in many of his post cancer treatment patients BP/IC symptoms. His thought was because of chemotherapy and/or radiation to the pelvic area the bladder lining cell division is changed and bladder-lining thinning over time becomes a big issue; this becomes post cancer treatment IC.

With the urologist I discussed an off label (not FDA approved) protection plan. The dosage of oral Elmiron would be increased before and during all the cancer treatment times to three Elmiron capsules in the morning and three in the evening. When radiation was scheduled I would stop first at the urology office and have an Elmiron bladder instillation with sterile saline put into to my bladder with a pediatric catheter and then I would head for the hospital to have my abdomen irradiated. Something worked because five years later my bladder bas been the least of my health problems.

Medicine is finally coming out of the dark ages for recognizing that lives may be spared with cancer treatments, but what happens to the body afterward changes how we live our lives. The word chronic covers many post cancer treatment conditions including bowel and bladder lining changes. My mountain to climb now is intestinal, large and small, because chemotherapy and radiation has changed how my bowels work forever.

The times I remember my bladder sending pain spasm signals was after potassium IV's I needed to bring my electrolytes back into balanced after multiple diarrhea episodes. I had lidocaine bladder instillations and ice packs to see me through those tough hours.

I shared with Jo that I never ask God why until this past year when after two lung operations for the removal of tumors, cancer was once again found in my lungs. Then I remembered the years of smoking and had my answer.

Five years has passed since that last cigarette, there has been the need for more surgery, radiation, and continuing chemotherapy as the cancer traveled to the outside of my bladder wall, pubic bone, and lungs. That is my heath reality news. The good life news is that I am still here and living each new day.

What I think

My health perspective is more intense than most of you hopefully will ever experience. The following is what I think after five years of hands on learning about my medical care in Southern California. Jo says I am working on my PhD in medicine. My hope is that no matter what phase of searching for answers and/or healing you are that some of my thoughts will help.

1. Needlepoint wisdom "God gives us only what we handle." I did wonder about the insight of that saying since my long list of health problems have been concentrated in this five year block of time; in fact my IC symptoms and concerns became the ground floor of dealing with what was going to occur with aggressive cancer treatments. There were multiple times when I wondered if I was going to find a way out of the jungle of pain, immense fatigue, multiple emergency rooms visits, hospital stays, medications, insurance forms, unsettled financial matters, family needs, and a stream of meeting personalities from helpful to hurtful, but it was all part of what is a learning curve. I think back to the "ah-ha" moments and how from every event you can learn.

2. Stop struggling. There are some things you cannot change, but how you react to them you can control. A nurse told me to think of a palm tree and how it bends even in the worst wind but does to snap. I have visualized that palm tree many, many times – it helps. At this writing my Dad and I are caring for my Mom, eighty two, whose dementia has continued to remove her from family life faster than her spreading breast cancer; I can't make her well, but I (we) have the choice to bend with demands of our joint need for care and ask for help.

3. Read the walls: Read what is posted on the office and exam room walls, i.e. letters, awards, diplomas, and posted notices. This is how I discovered that in California there is a financial support program "Hospital Financial Screening Assessment Form"; if you earn less than 23,000 dollars a year there is help for medical and medication bills.

4. Keep all your records, reports, and test results discs in a three ring binder-a two inch one (resource-Costco package of 3) – and request copies of all your reports. Your medical records belong to you. If you gather them with each visit you will have a logical record of your care. The Lance Armstrong Foundation is still a great resource, and has binder organizer to help with keeping track of the multiple appointments and tests.

5. Keep a calendar. The calendar whether paper or electronic keeps you sane. My cell phone located list of appointments, medication, documents due, checks to arrive, etc. reduced confusion when stress should be minimal. I started keeping track of records and appointments when I began taking my IC treatment seriously and that helped me to communicate from one heath care source to another and not make appointment mistakes.

6. Look beyond the IC diet to stabilize your digestive system. Investigate the use of probiotic such as the product, Align. A GI physician who also has bowel problems brought this product to my attention. After many courses of antibiotics, surgical, and medical treatments, and diarrhea became brutal and compromised my very life. I am now on a special routine that balances diet and medication.

7. High fiber foods and supplements may make the bowel situation worse. Inflammation causes IC flares and can often coincide with bowel irritation and diarrhea. Wheat (gluten) can also be a trigger.

8. Keep away from greasy foods. Two items that work are extra virgin olive oil (EVO) and if needed paper towels to soak up grease. I use both to assure that I have the least amount of grease in my diet. When my bowels are settled my bladder is also quiet.

9. Stress reduction: Often part of the discussion but as often a struggle to achieve. My choice was Rieki therapy, the Japanese art of stress reduction and promotion of healing. I went to therapy sessions at my local hospital, during a particularly difficult time it was very helpful.

10. Find your voice; the most difficult for most of us to accomplish and yet the key for me of recovery from whatever life lays at our doorstep. I remember listening to the cancer treatment plans and not understanding how in the world it would relate to me. I found the courage to look up 5-FU (Fluorouracil), found it has been used in treatment since 1958, and began to understand why it was the chemotherapy of choice for me. Because of that understanding I started my cancer recovery with less anxiety.

What seems like a lifetime ago I discovered that recovery from IC meant not a cure but control and containment of runaway symptoms. That very same recovery model guides me today, as I know that my tumor sites require effort to control and contain their growth. What I think is that another meaning of recovery is renewal and suddenly it is a new day. I wish you the best.

11.

Donna, age 58
IC Symptoms Have Changed My Life

Background

Donna is 58 years old, divorced. She has two grown daughters, age 36 and 40, six grandkids, ages six to 16. She was born in Poplar Bluff, Missouri, the youngest of ten. Her parents brought them all to California when she was just 2 years old. She was married and pregnant at seventeen. Her first-born daughter was nine pounds six ounces and twenty-two inches long; second daughter was not quite so large. Both are wonderful young woman who share Donna's joy of life.

Donna's Story

I had very good grades in school and was very active with the student body. I was treasurer in the seventh grade, vice president in the eighth grade, and in the ninth grade was president. Good grades and my high energy launched me into being both a class officer and cheerleader in high school. I can remember trying out for cheer and after practice being the only person running to the restroom to empty my bladder. I did not have any pain, just had to visit the restroom a lot.

My discovery is that since childhood I have made life adjustments for urinary symptoms, without connecting frequent voiding and the progression to pelvic pain as the reflection of my bladder lining being unable to protect me from the acid effects of urine. My story is how I took all the clues and began to make sense out of how my life has been changed because of Interstitial Cystitis.

I am self-employed due to my IC. I did not realize how the act of peeing was going to control my future when it started out with my *just* using the restroom more often, especially after coffee, but frankly that did not strike me as unusual since caffeine and more trips to the bathroom go hand in hand. Because I was working in a corporate office, as an administrative assistant for the Vice President of real estate, I was lucky to have a restroom close by; the only problem was we had to use a key to open the restroom. I learned to always carry the key with me. This was a clue that my need to void was greater than others. If you had told me that my bladder was going to impact my future I would have thought you were joking.

As I look back, I know that as a young girl I always had to use the restroom more often than others. I wet the bed until I was 6 years old. Lucky for me, my mom never once got on me; she would just strip the bed and wash the sheets. That says a lot about my Mom, who had ten children and I was number ten. I did not have pain then as I do now. I did notice that I would need to empty my bladder more around the time when my period was due. I was fortunate not to have bad menstrual cramps or long periods. The cycle of the serious need to pee was always there.

As a young mother, I knew the usual story of children stopping all forward motion as they need to go to the restroom that brings family travel to a halt. I remember taking vacations when my daughters were young; we would always stop because I was the one who needed to use the restroom, not them.

When I was married I did get a few bladder infections after sexual intercourse and occasionally sex would be painful. My husband was not circumcised and the thought was that intercourse brought about bladder infections because of the bacteria from his penis. My urine was sent out for culture and I remember once having to go to the emergency room because the bladder pain was so overwhelming; the diagnosis was infection. All that being said, my pelvic pain seemed at times to be greater during sex and after intercourse the urge to pee was even stronger.

Did pelvic distress lead to issues with my marriage? I have to answer yes with the explanation that my husband was so young and he just didn't get it. As I recall for the most part sex was not bad because I learned the positions that didn't hurt.

I was 48 when the real bladder problems started. My pelvic pain was intense. Because of my history of bladder infections I made a direct connection that the urge, frequency, and pain were caused once again by bacteria. I went to the doctor and the medical office always found blood in my urine. I do not know if they sent my urine specimens to the lab, because no infection was reported, yet I was still prescribed antibiotics.

One day, I was in so much pain at work, I had to be driven home and was put on two weeks of medical leave. I was sent to an urologist and they could not figure out what I had. When I went back to work I was told I no longer had a job. I couldn't afford the optional COBRA medical insurance, so I went without coverage; that stopped all medical care. I had to make a big adjustment in how I was going to continue my life.

Being unemployed did not stop the pelvic pain. I think the stress of wondering what was going to happen next in my life brought on earthquake flares. I remember locking myself in my room for days because I hurt so much. My gynecologist referred me to another urologist. That urologist did not have any answers. They were going to do some tests, but because of my not having any insurance the tests were never done. I did see a doctor who was a friend's recommendation. He did not give me any reason for my bladder symptoms but recommended that I stay away from red pasta sauces and spicy foods because he said these particular diet choices were probably irritating my bladder. I had to pay cash for that visit and advice.

One time, a nurse brought a form to me that asked questions like, "Are you depressed and do you want to kill yourself?" I remember thinking what the heck is this all about - I am a happy person who had unexplained pelvic pain and my unhappiness was the frustration directed to not knowing what was going wrong. My concern is how the depression labels are thrown around by the medical profession because the reason for a condition cannot be pinned down. IC has no basic test and that makes for confusion, frustration, and anger.

I went back to work; this time I am self-employed and work from my home mostly on the computer and I am right next to the bathroom. Some days can be so frustrating because I will have to pee six times in an hour. I have to stop what I am doing and then find my place again with typing. Sometimes when I receive a phone call I try to make sure I answer the cordless phone because I have had to actually use the bathroom during the conversation. Not so much fun. There are days when the bladder symptoms are not as bad because I have watched what I have eaten the week before. Food is key.

I started my own research online. I spent hours typing in my bladder symptoms and reading everything I could about pelvic pain. I finally came to the conclusion that IC was a front-runner for what was causing my recurring misery. Armed with renewed health insurance, I made an appointment with an urologist near my home and he went over my symptoms and agreed that my story of urge, frequency, and pelvic pain probably was IC. I asked how could we know for sure and he commented that there was one procedure that might confirm that I had IC, a cystoscopy. I said I wanted it done. Until I asked directly for the test, he wasn't going to order it and was going to let me leave with the question of the reason for my bladder pain unanswered.

When the cystoscopy finally was done, I got my answer. It was IC. From that diagnosis point I was prescribed Elmiron and was left on my own. I continued under this urologist care for about a year and found I was not getting any better. I went back online and found Dr. Davis, who was very familiar with IC. It has been about eight years since I made an appointment and my life began to change for the better because I found a urology office that gave me information to guide me in expanding my time for staying pain free and rescues for the days when my IC roars.

A major issue I encountered was the need to void and not being able to because of blockage in the urethra. I did not know why at first and then found out it was a blood clot from my bladder lining that was beyond inflammation; it was ulcerated and bleeding. The first time this inability to void happened the pelvic pain was so excruciating that the paramedics were called. I passed the clot before they arrived but the bleeding from my bladder was the symptom that pointed directly to a bladder lining ulceration that had compromised my health even more.

What is labeled Hunner's Ulcers is what has so compromised my bladder lining, the ulcer causes spontaneous bleeding and emergency measures have to be taken. I have had these frightening bleed episodes a number of times and I have learned to have catheters in my possession if I need to push past the clot to remove urine from my bladder. I know with IC, blood clots are not the only reason that a catheter might be needed to remove urine from the bladder. The bladder can become so spastic because of irritation that a person cannot void. This is when having a tube put in your bladder to remove urine is a needed rescue. I use a brand of plastic catheter called LoFric; it is made from plastic so not to start any allergic reaction. I have learned to stay away from all latex items for the strong possibility that I will have an allergic response and make a bad situation even worse; hospital emergency rooms as a general rule continue to use latex catheters so I have my own. The LoFric catheter when in contact with water has a very slick coating and women's' size of 8 or 10 French (sizing standard) keeps the chance of injury when inserted less likely. I have also learned how to position myself on the toilet so the pain will be alleviated.

I have had another cystoscopy to check for bladder cancer, because blood in the urine can mean a bacterial infection, ulceration, stone, and cancer, and needs to be checked. I have made changes in my diet as less acidic foods and I had a series of bladder instillations of

Elmiron. I was doing the bladder instillations with Elmiron and lidocaine but unfortunately I found it was too hard for me to hold the medication and any value of coating my bladder with direct contact was lost. What I have learned is to develop a roster of rescues and treatment information. I gained a sense of some control to move ahead with my life and not keep spinning in place.

Before I go further with my story I want to recommend being part of a clinical trial. I have been involved in clinical trials about IC. One was about coating the bladder directly with the use of a catheter using Elmiron, another was about pelvic pain control. First, you will find a more involved standard of medical care that is focused on a specific problem; for me it was pelvic pain caused by IC. You are involved with people that understand your condition and share new information along the way. Also the trial information might help you get better. Most of all you are helping the next group of women fighting their battles with IC. Downsides for me included a long drive, but it was worth it.

IC has changed my life. I am a person that loves living a high-energy style, simply described as go, go, and go even more. IC has shortened my activity list as life continues to revolve around the need to be near restroom facilities. For a long time, lifting my grandbabies has been scratched from my "can do list." When the IC symptoms hit my life I had to change from running to walking because bouncing hurt. I use to love to take my grandson to the park and go down the slide with him; we would play baseball and softball and I would play soccer with my granddaughter. My family has always had big picnics and I would be the first in line to play. The great hurt is the need to limit my activities, yet I have learned to enjoy sharing other interests with them. I would not be telling the truth if I said that the substitutions are the perfect answer to what I have missed but accommodations had to be made so I could be participate in my grandchildren's lives. The modifications are worth it.

Exercise has always been brought a feeling of wellbeing into my life. With bladder lining inflammation and pelvic pain this was limited to wishing I could return to my workouts. There was a time that I could no longer run on a treadmill. That was a dark time. As of today, I go to the gym three times a week and I am back for my walks on the treaded mill. I have started lifting weights again: and caution everyone to take it slowly and know that it is repetitions that build the tone and strength not the number of pounds. I do notice that if I do a lot of bending I can bring on bladder pain. As a counter to that discomfort I find that stretching and deep breathing seems to help bring my mind and body back to center. And I can tell you my very favorite is a very warm bath that allows my muscles to relax and the pain to go down the drain.

I also have to say no to my friends when they want to go boating unless there is a bathroom aboard. Boating is an example of a reason to join friends and enjoy a special lunch; there I am with my lettuce. I do know that one of my relationships ended when the man I was seeing wanted to visit Mazatlán. He loved to travel but even in neighboring Mexico my food choices were limited and the joy of travel and our association ended. IC symptoms have changed my life.

The most important lesson I have learned is that the food we eat plays the largest role of all in maintaining a pelvic zone that is pain free. When I follow the IC diet, I almost feel normal, *almost* being a key word in that statement. If I stray from my diet rules I can feel the discomfort and bladder pain again. I love chocolate so much that at times reach for the Godiva and know I will pay with pelvic pain. I know that Motrin and baking soda will be my rescue of choice. My motto is you have to live your life.

My daughter does most of the cooking and she has learned so much about IC, beginning with the separation of the meat to be prepared so that the family has it marinated and mine is not. When she makes tacos, she will set my organic ground beef aside for me before she seasons the rest for the family. When I eat at a restaurant and have something as simple as chicken soup, I have experienced some degree of pelvic pain, at home, with my own prepared food; I am safer from these negative experiences. I love avocado and will use it instead of mayonnaise, even the avocado will give me a twinge of pain but I can handle it and it passes. I do know that bananas affect me and if I crave them, I will take just a few bites so not to push the pain button. Most packaged cereals will bring on a negative effect as well. Every now and then I will go ahead and try a new approach, like I love yogurt so lately I have been having Greek yogurt from Trader Joe's and my bladder lining does not seem to mind. Maybe that is the main dietary lesson: Just because a food is in the do not eat column for IC, we are all individuals and need to find out what works for us.

I do buy true organic when possible. I can eat eggs, bread, potatoes, and most all meats seasoned with salt an a little pepper. Vegetables cause me no problems. I usually bake chicken and grill steak. I steam my veggies with a small amount of butter. I have eaten standard chicken (not organic) and have been O.K. I prepare most of my foods and stay away from foods that have been prepared because of the additives and preservatives because I do not want to risk how my body will react to the unknown ingredients. I realize that I have food sensitivities that bring on bladder reactions.

I do notice a small flare when I eat a whole banana or try what is supposed to be a safe soft drink like root beer. It seems that within two hours I feel my negative choice has brought about increased bladder lining inflammation or it can creep up on me and later in the evening I will know I have strayed from the IC diet path.

When at a restaurant I have learned to ask if the meat is marinated because then I know I can't eat it. Then I ask them to use olive oil when grilling. I will ask for a baked potato with butter on the side and salad without dressing. I did learn that at one restaurant their grilled zucchini was rubbed with vinegar, so asking how food is prepared is a smart move. For the most part, I have found restaurant personal very understanding after I explain that I am dealing with health issues. I simply say I have a bladder problem and if I eat the wrong things I am in extreme pain. I say that I am not picky about food, my bladder is.

What I Think

1. I can't emphasize enough that reading all the information you can about IC.

2. The Interstitial Cystitis Association (ICA) should be pushing for a test for IC. Physicians rarely think about the connection of bladder pain to IC. The norm is to continue to hand us a prescription for an antibiotic.

3. Most important is to find a doctor who understands IC and cares. If I had found a more knowledgeable Doctor early on, it would have saved me much pain and suffering.

4. Again I say learn as much as you can about what foods triggers your pain, which is good place to start.

5. Diet is often the last item that is recognized as an influence in IC. I think it is more than 50% for control of symptoms.

6. If the medical profession recognized that IC is real and understood the life changing impact of pelvic pain, this would be a true break through for us all.

7. Learn relaxation techniques, I know it is easier to say and harder to do, but the feeling of being over whelmed can take all body pain to a higher level. Practice the techniques of quieting your pain demons before pain becomes overwhelming.

8. When you begin to improve discuss with your physician any changes in your medication regimen. Often the wonderful stable period of less pelvic pain goes off the tracks because the lining of the bladder always needs protection and genetically speaking, I know I do not make the needed cells.

9. I am one person who tried to go off Elmiron because I thought it wasn't helping. I began to return to my more pelvic pain state and more frequent visits to the restrooms; when I would eat something not on the IC safe list the pain was more intense. That is why I think any change you make in your medicine, be cautious and do not shrug off increased symptoms.

10. IC does not go away. I think of it as an allergic response to a bladder lining that does not heal well. Stronger symptoms are a signal that I have to be more careful.

12. Arianne's Story, age 49
My Story

My name is Arianne, age 49, and I have been married 28 years to a loving and supportive man. I have four children ranging in ages from 13 to 26. I have been a teacher of young children when not raising little ones of my own. I am very involved in my church, garden for enjoyment, exercise, and spend most of time doing family-oriented activities.

I grew up happy and healthy, raised on home-cooked meals made from fresh ingredients. I was taught good nutrition habits and to avoid preservatives. My life was basically ideal for years into my early adulthood.

Looking back, something changed after my third pregnancy, when our child was stillborn. I was 25 and had two normal pregnancies, but this time a placental abruption resulted in five trips to the hospital, invasive procedures (i.e. catheterization) and strong medicines to attempt to stop early contractions. After this experience my physical sexual response was a little different, but my gynecologist denied a problem. As years passed, I would regularly mention that I had some irritation during sex, however he claimed everything was fine. I also began to feel a pressure on my abdomen during sex. It was not exactly painful, but uncomfortable. My husband and I went to get counseling, because I started to think the issues were in my head. Through the therapist I was directed to a uro-gynecologist who diagnosed me with a very irritated genital track. My husband got a vasectomy; birth control creams were definitely exaggerating the problem. I seem to be sensitive/allergic to them and they caused the irritation and some of the discomfort.

However, part of the pain remained and I experienced the pain as pressure, burning, and lower back pain. My doctor at the time began diagnosing me with urinary tract infections. He always did a dipstick test of my urine, but usually started me on antibiotics before sending the specimen to the lab. Because of my continued discomfort, my doctor concluded that I had urethritis and prescribed urethral dilations to open up the urethra and reduce pain. These were handled in the office with no anesthesia. I had only two of these treatments because they were excruciatingly painful and neither helped me physically, nor psychologically.

This uro-gynecologist also prescribed physical therapy with a specialist that used internal muscle release and biofeedback. This might have been very helpful, as years of pain had caused me to develop pelvic floor muscle spasms. It was an odd experience, but the therapist was careful to protect my modesty as much as possible. She was friendly and matter of fact about the process. However, I continued to consume lemonade and other acidic foods unaware of what was really happening in my body, so I experienced only minor, intermittent relief.

Throughout my experiences, I have dealt with a deep sadness over the slow loss of my sexuality. My husband has been patient and loving and faithful during a time when many men would have given up. I have attempted to meet his needs when, at times, my heart was breaking over my inability to feel the level of pleasure, joy and closeness that sex once gave me.

After five years of treatment, one day my pain did not reduce with two different courses of antibiotics. My uro-gynecologist finally shared with me that he had concluded that I had interstitial cystitis. It seemed that he was reluctant to diagnose me because it was difficult to confirm and there were few available treatment options. He prescribed Elmiron and Elavil and suggested some diet changes and referred me to a holistic doctor that tried to help determine the allergy connection. I was found to have so many allergies that if I followed his diet restrictions; I could find little to eat.

In my search to discover what IC was, I ran across a local support group and attended a meeting. That led me to an urologist who conducted research in the field and was current on the latest treatment options. I have tried all different combinations of nerve pain medicines (Elavil, Neurontin, and Lyrica), antihistamines (Benadryl, Allegra), muscle relaxants, and Elmiron in order to be comfortable with varying degrees of success. When I am at my worst, I will try any combination of these drugs to get by.

I saw Elmiron as the only means of "healing" my bladder. However, I took it for two years without really seeing a direct improvement. I also had instillations at the doctor's office without noticeable results. Elmiron eventually took its toll on my body. I began having loose stools and finally such bad problems that I couldn't always get to the bathroom in time. It was becoming debilitating. My colonoscopy revealed intestines that were a "friable mucosa" or irritated to point of fragility. My colon was so damaged that my doctor could not complete the procedure because he feared tearing through the tissue. Upon the suggestion of my gastroenterologist, I stopped taking Elmiron. Clearly I suffered from some of the possible side effects because, without the drug, my digestive system healed over the next few months and I was much improved in this respect.

Recently, I started having new symptoms, which prevented me from sleeping at night. Once again, I was having abdominal pain that was difficult to describe. After many thorough tests, my gastroenterologist suggested that I go off of gluten (wheat, etc.) since an endoscopy indicated a possible allergy to it. Some relief occurred over the next few weeks. In general my digestive system is much more regular which in turn helps my IC symptoms. Whenever some part of me is stirred up in the pelvic region, my bladder is not happy. In retrospect, I wonder how long I had had these abdominal symptoms combined with the other symptoms causing confusion for my doctors and me.

There is some evidence at this point that my bladder has healed significantly. My uro-gynecologist looked at it recently while performing a cystoscopy and indicated as much. Now, I can "cheat" with small amounts of IC-sensitive foods if I space out the consumption over days. It is clear to me now that I cannot comfortably eat gluten. However, with all of this improvement, my pubic area nerves are still almost always "up-regulated." I cannot get them to calm down completely even when I am otherwise virtually symptom-free. I will have an itchy feeling when the discomfort is mild and more of a burning feeling as the pain increases. I have experienced relief with medication, but it continues to affect my sexual response.

I started going to a support group shortly after my diagnosis and it has been helpful. I am educated on the latest information and research about IC. I get specific suggestions about lifestyle changes that I can make and it is nice to know that I am not alone in my physical struggles. I feel like my pain is validated, that I am not crazy and that others understand what I am going through.

What I think:
1. I am in charge of my body, my life.

2. Medicine is not all science. Everyone's body is different with its own mysteries and delicate balance of chemicals, hormones,

emotions and physical issues. We have to learn about ourselves, and advocate for our health needs.

3. Physicians seem to only know about their own specialty these days. Our body's systems overlap; therefore we have to be the bridge between our doctors.

4. It is helpful to ask for a copy of every test a doctor performs and keep those in a folder, along with notes about their recommendations, drugs prescribed, and changes that have been helpful. You will avoid repeating tests and delaying treatment because of a lack of detailed information.

5. Doctors mean well, but they are not perfect. Analyze their suggestions and use your good judgment. Get second and third and fourth opinions. A good doctor will tell you when he has exhausted his ability to help you. He will lead you to additional resources.

6. Try not to give in to depression. Difficult times last for a season. If you hang in there, it will get better.

7. Do not let a physical issue destroy your relationships. It is natural to get irritable, frustrated, or sad when you don't feel well. I found this especially true before having a clear diagnosis. However, try to set the pain aside as much as possible. Just because you have been dealt a secret pain doesn't mean everyone around you has to suffer as well.

8. Let little things in life go when you are not feeling well (a perfectly cleaned house, home-made cookies, driving on a field trip). Eventually you will be able to do more again.

9. Let your spouse be a partner in your health care. Ask for help running errands or taking care of children, ask for a backrub, and ask for a shoulder to cry on sometimes. However, don't overburden him with discouraging details because you will need his bright outlook to keep you going. Remember that even if you are struggling sexually, he has normal healthy feelings that need to be met. He especially needs to know that you still love him and are not rejecting him even during the times when you are unable to enjoy sex.

10. Pray for wisdom and guidance as you seek help. Ask God for strength and patience as you deal with a difficult disease. Be thankful each day for all the blessings that you do have. Learn a new empathy for those who also suffer every day as they deal with their own health issues, carrying the burden of a secret pain.

13. Kristine E., age 25
My Journey for Answers

My name is Kristine, and I'm 25 years old. I needed to learn about my health and to deal with health problems at an early age; this situation was caused by the demands of a series of health events topped off by pelvic pain. The learning experience of having my lower abdomen wrapped by pelvic pain is not a choice I would have made yet these circumstances have helped me mature in many ways. This is my story.

In my family, I've never heard or seen any other family member who has had to deal with pelvic pain. My sister is sensitive to certain foods, but usually it only affects her skin. So the medical label of interstitial cystitis was very new to my family and me. I continue to learn and teach them. It is an ongoing experience.

As a child I remember I always needed to use the restroom a lot. At sleepovers, I would be embarrassed to have to get up so many times at night to use the restroom. At that age you don't realize you have a problem because it seems like something so ordinary.

When I was in 10 years old I was in the car and needed to use the restroom and my mom didn't want to pull over and I ended up not being able to hold it because it hurt too much. After that, I never wanted to make a big deal of my bathroom habits because I felt ashamed. When I came into my teenage years, around 16 and 17 years old, is when I started getting frequent bladder infections. My friends would get them every so often so I never thought too much of it. After I graduated high school, I would get sharp pain down in my abdominal area. I would go to see different doctors and it seemed no one would take the time to figure out what is wrong with me. I was finally sent to get an ultra sound where I had up to four or five golf ball sized cysts on each ovary. The pain became so bad that it was caused me to miss work and other functions. People thought I was just trying to get out of work and being lazy.

The last three years is when my symptoms started to show more often. Being the age I am, I would go out with friends and have alcoholic drinks but be in pain for the next 3 days afterwards. This occurred every time I drank. It made me want to stay in bed all day. Then the allergies came. I have never been allergic to anything in my life and it was strange to me how all of a sudden I couldn't be around dust or a cat without having a major asthma attack.

The symptoms continued and the pain became more constant. I knew something was wrong. After seeing my gynecologist who simply said "Having pain is part of being a female, so we just have to deal with it". She then sent me to another gynecologist who pretty much said the same thing. I decided to go see my regular physician who suggested I do full blood work and another ultra sound. After the results for those painful experiences came back, they found nothing! The pain continued to get worse and I was having vaginal bleeding almost every day. My gynecologist still didn't believe anything was wrong with me. She finally sent me to a nearby urologist to "check my bladder". The doctor came into the office asked me some questions and told me to go on Elmiron. I took it 3 times a day everyday along with instillation treatments 3 times a week for 3 weeks. They used a "red robin" that is a catheter made of rubber that caused me so much pain I cried every time. The nurses would mess up each time and have to redo the procedure a couple times or have multiple nurses to help assist. It was painful, humiliating and embarrassing. That doctor never showed her face again. I was sent for full body CT scans twice and more blood work, again, nothing. My gynecologist finally sent me to another urologist about 2 hours away who stuck a large needle into my abdomen and poked up and down and asked me where it hurt. At this point endometriosis was brought up but was said to be unlikely because of my age. I was beginning to feel hopeless.

When I hit a wall of abdominal pain, narcotic medication was a lifeline; but what seems like a solution becomes a greater problem to overcome. The medication side effects made me ill and I just wanted the pain to be over. I know that you who are reading this understand the pain and despair that can sweep away all thoughts. The pain medication became my way to numb the pain and my feelings towards everything. Simple Advil would not work anymore so I was prescribed Vicodin by my family doctor. After that stopped working came the Oxytocin, and the doses becoming higher and higher. This was just the band aid covering my problem.

At this point my emotions where out of control. I was frustrated and angry. I didn't know who or what to be angry at, so I blamed myself. Doctors have told me they don't know the cause of IC or BPS, but I suffered from a serious eating disorder for 13 years and feel that could have been the cause of my problems. I would cry a lot, more out of frustration then from depression. I wanted to sleep most days but I had to work. My work suffered, my family suffered and I had to take a leave of absence from school.

My eating disorder was a five-year period spent not eating, starving myself to control my weight. I started to binge on food and make myself throw-up, three to four times a day. I began to have hair loss and loss of the enamel of on my teeth and both stomach and lower abdominal pain. Now in my early twenties I have slowly stopped this destructive behavior but still have times when I slip back into old patterns of threating my body as an enemy.

I started to think that this was just going to be my life forever and I won't ever be normal again. To have my life turned upside down over night was taking a toll on me. That was until I came across a woman to who came into my work and over heard me talking to my co-worker about my symptoms. She told me she had the same ones and recommended a doctor that was close by. I knew I was hitting a dead end so I gave them a try. After attending a support group meeting, my hopes were brought back up. I made an appointment and the urologist knew from my symptoms something had to be done as soon as possible. I was scared and happy and just mentally exhausted after everything to have someone finally say, "I can help you." Those words saved me.

The day of my surgery I was calm and ready. I never felt happier to be at a hospital. The cystoscopy and laparoscopy were performed at the same time. When I came out of surgery my doctor came to me, and the first thing he said was, "we found the endometriosis and removed it, and you also have interstitial cystitis." If I had not just come out of surgery I would have been jumping for joy, not because I have it but because I now knew what was going on. Things were going to be different.

I knew my life would have to change. I just didn't know how drastic the change would be. Even before I knew I had IC for sure I was trying to make changes in my life. The diet has been the hardest for me. Not being able to open the refrigerator and eating whatever I felt like was frustrating. My family has tried to work around my new dietary habits and I feel like it's my fault they have to make or do something separate because of me. It becomes harder and harder to try to explain to someone how this feels and have them understand. You find yourself feeling very alone. Not only do we hurt physically but mentally as well. I would love to sleep the whole night for once. I would love to feel energized throughout the day. I would love to go a whole day without any kind of medication. And I would love to have a normal relationship with someone. The emotional stress can sometimes take it toll. When it comes down to it, I feel every IC'er needs a support group to go to, a good doctor and plenty of water to help balance everything.

When it comes to food, drinks and medications, I have been educating myself a lot. Knowing the small details can make the difference. I know to stay away from tomatoes, onions, pineapple (and juices), champagne, beer, spicy food and anything with magnesium. Those are probably my top "bad" things I know will cause a flare within 24 hours or less. Controlling my diet has made the biggest difference in how many and how long my flares will last. When I switched to a gluten free diet, not only did my bladder feel better, but my whole body did as well. I never have been a big caffeine person, so I don't miss it. I do drink peppermint tea with a little honey that makes me feel better. When I prepare my own meals I know what's being put in so I don't risk the chance of any preservatives or citric acid. You can still make a good tasteful dinner with out all of the "bad" things. I was recommended an IC cookbook and that has helped me and my family a lot. And I always bring my own snacks and lunch to work. Having carrot sticks, celery, almonds and granola bars stocked always helps. And my number one "good" thing to have is water (spring) with you wherever you go. I know we try to avoid it because of the frequent bathroom use, but water helps dilute our pee so the pressure and pain is decreased.

Exercising is also on the good list. I used to love to run. The pain made it hard to even walk sometimes and made exercising almost non-existent. I have found that a light walk and yoga type stretching makes a huge difference with my muscles and relaxation techniques. After exercising or from walking a lot, I love to use heating pads or soak in a warm bath. Heat has always been the better choice for me to relax and ease pain. The recommendation is for ice packs to reduce the inflammation and therefore the pain; my use of heat to reduce pain points out that that IC is a very personal disorder.

Even though I don't know where my IC and endometriosis came from or how they will be cured, I know that I need to be involved in becoming educated and making the changes in my life style that make sense to me. I started learning about both diseases. With help from my doctor and help from others diagnosed, I was able to realize how important it is to understand my body and how IC has effected it. I wanted to help others and help them learn as I did. I started reaching out by having my story put in a newspaper article and had a positive response from people who have been in the dark about IC. Soon I was helping with online support chats and social networking groups. I also helped by public speaking to others who suffer as I do. I realized that I would never help myself by lying in bed all day not knowing what to do. Someone with IC can live a normal life. I hope to have a successful relationship with someone who cares about me, not my IC. I hope to be able to have a child one day if possible. And one day, I hope to do the things IC has been holding me back from. But hope is just an expected wish. I don't expect anything to happen to me unless I move forward with my plans. My educational goal is that I have returned to school and am working on becoming a sign language interpreter. Returning to school was the first step to taking back my life.

What I know

I have found that dealing with so many doctors and medications that having IC is not easy. It's day-by-day process that will sometimes be harder on most days then others. For me:

1. If I'm tired I rest or take a nap. We need it.

2. Following the low acid diet

3. Having a travel case of extra medications, heating pads, comfortable underwear and pants and travel water bottle.

4. Taking vitamins E, D, A and selenium to boost my immune system.

5. Find the right antihistamine, for night and for day.

6. Going to a support group meeting.

7. Don't be afraid to ask questions. Write them down and keep track of flares.

8. I go pee as soon as I feel it. Even if it irritates me, it's worse in the long run to hold it.

9. Don't be afraid to cry.

10. Be honest about your pelvic pain with other people. At times it is the most difficult to explain to family, friends, and a girl or boy friend. I have used descriptive terms for my body's response to bladder's inflammation as an allergic response, sunburn, and a muscle injury like an athletic would experience.

14. Eva, age 77
My Heath and History

Background

"Many, many bladder infections from the age of ten," that is how Eva, now seventy-seven, answered the question about urinary problem in childhood. Born in Germany, Eva became a US citizen in 1966. She is a mother of two sons, and grandmother to four. After fifty-four years of marriage, Eva had to adjust her life to a husband in rapidly declining health and recently, widowhood. The past four years have been filled with multiple life changes. Eva's continued search for pelvic pain recovery is proof that with age comes wisdom and health problems are there as the part of reality of being human. Her story has the revelation of a childhood with the extraordinary stress of World War II that few will ever experience.

Eva's Story

When I reached the age of 75 I found myself a widow. I became aware that an entire new life was about to develop for me, not by choice but because I am the survivor of a long marriage. My reoccurring question was if my Bladder Pain Syndrome/Interstitial Cystitis (BPS/IC) was going to hold me back from completing all the decisions and tasks that came with the death of my husband and would BPS/IC limit how I would move forward with my life?" The answer is that after a difficult and question filled three months I was determined to move forward.

I am a woman who by nature is reserved, but I do come directly to the point and say the truth as I have experienced it. BPS/IC linked to the word chronic gave me the reason for years of pelvic pain; BPS/IC took away my sense of good health and sexual pleasure. My search for the reason for the pelvic pain was shorter than most, but the years of growing distance between my husband and me is a sadness that is mine.

But I am getting ahead of myself; let me start my story in 1955 when I left Germany and moved to Canada. I worked at a bank in Germany and an associate had moved to Canada in 1954. He changed my life's direction by sending me the money to relocate. But Sault Ste Marie is very cold and in 1961 after marriage to Wilfred and the birth of two sons the family moved to southern California. We were so fortunate to find our first home in Ontario and we have lived in the same area all these years.

My husband was an accountant and was motivated to go to night school and achieve certification as an auditor/CPA and a lawyer. His business expertise was a blessing because the choices made at the time of his retirement from Southern Californian Edison have impacted our and now my medical care. Given todays confused, chaotic insurance choices and financial constraints as to when or if you can go to a medical specialist I continue to be fortunate. My husband, as he was at the point of retirement, was given a choice of retiring at 62 with medical benefits for life or retiring at 65 with financial compensation. He chose the health insurance benefit. I write this to point out that the intensity of our joint medical demands was a continuing rolling thunderstorm for me; for my husband it was a tornado as he fought cancer. Both our health needs demanded more with each passing year and I have appreciated his wisdom in choosing the best insurance coverage when retiring at 62.

I also know that I am fortunate to have the choice of medical care because part of the recovery from BPS/IC is the vigilance needed to make sure if urinary urgency and frequency increases that bacteria is not the cause of or part of the bladder's inflammation problem; this means a trip to the doctor's office and a urine specimen sent to the laboratory for a culture and sensitivity. The results, if positive, gives the physician the identity of the bacteria involved and the appropriate antibiotic for treatment; if negative, that conclusion also requires a medical evaluation and for me to deal with the source of the inflammation that often is traced to stress, food choices, or seasonal allergies. When these join together to produce my bladder's increased pain, recovery often needs professional medical direction and care and that means medical cost.

Some people ask how IC affected my family dynamics. I must answer by saying we did not talk about it. The frustration grew when I tried to explain how urgency, frequency, and getting up to the bathroom two and three times a night does not make for a great frame of mind; my words fell on deaf ears. In fact I felt that somehow it was my fault for experiencing the pelvic ache that would make me feel so hopeless.

This is what happened to me as I looked for a reason for my pelvic pain and numerous trips to the bathroom. Ten years ago I opened the phone book and found by the luck of a number Dr. Davis's office. That act of going to an urologist started me on the journey to take better care of myself and directed me to the purpose of actively looking for answers to control my IC. He understood my problem, not every doctor does.

One question was whether my husband understood my bladder pain; the answer was *sometimes*. He did come with me to some of the IC Support meetings but men as a general rule and my husband specifically want to fix the problems. The word chronic is not one that fits well in any relationship. His sense of control was challenged as my sense of control was compromised. It was a struggle.

I cannot tell you how many times stress whirled around my life and now I realize, for me, seventy five percent of my pelvic pain intensity was related to anxiety. It is sad to say, but I feel better since Will's death. I am still sad, yes, but my nerves and my bladder are much better. I do not know what the connection is, but when Dr. Davis addresses neuropathic pain, I appreciate what he is saying about how stress builds in power and feeds off itself. Now I am battling an irritable bowel (IBS) and wonder if any of you have had one chronic symptom become more troublesome than another?

At the Support Group we had a speaker who spoke about sensitivity to wheat or gluten, Celiac Disease. I know that often migraine, Fibromyalgia, and bowel irritably can add to the painful symptoms with IC. This knowledgeable woman addressed how after years of searching for a reason for her painful muscles that her sensitivity to wheat was discovered. She stated that the blood test for Celiac Disease (gluten sensitivity) is unreliable and the test of choice is genetic test from simple cotton swabbing from the inside of your mouth and sent to Kimball Genetics a Division of LabCorp a testing facility in Denver, Colorado.

I took the opportunity to have this test; my Medicare Insurance covered the cost but the results proved to be inconclusive. I decided because of my irritable bowel symptoms to try the gluten free diet. I went on a gluten free diet for four weeks and had no less symptoms of IC or irritable bowel. Now I have decided to eat not only nonacid foods but NO white bread, a little sugar, and raw carrots. It is a simple change to make and I am giving it a longer test.

IC aches and pains do not stop me from traveling to visit friends and relatives. This is a real joy in my life. I have a sister living Germany plus many uncles, aunts, cousins, and friends. I had the wonderful experience of having twenty phone calls from Germany on my recent birthday. I am going to visit there in the month of June for five weeks. I plan to go to what we call the old country that is Poland now. There I will go to the town of Breslau. I went to the boarding school there. I also would like to go to the place my grandparents loved. I had a wonderful and loving grandmother. She loved me so much more than my own mother. The memories mean so much to me

I also travel to Canada to visit very close friends and I plan on at least a three-week visit every year. I am looking forward to the Canadian trip and hosting a friend's 85th birthday party. I will be in a group of nine friends who have stayed in touch for over fifty years

This brings up the topic of travel and IC. These are some of my methods of making sure I have a do not have a crisis of IC symptoms when I am traveling. First I have a rescue kit that includes Pyridium (Phenozoyridine Hydrochloride) as a pain reliever for urinary tract irritation. I use this as a rescue and drink a lot of water to dilute my urine.

I have made many changes in my diet since I began this search for how to control my bladder pain and now the addition of bowel problems. First I have eliminated as much as I can of foods that are primarily have a high acid content like the often used example of raw tomatoes. Acid seems to be one of my main trigger foods for my bladder to tell me this was the wrong thing to eat or drink.

That is why the over the counter product, Prelief, helps an anti-acid diet along. I eat only pears, stay away from apples, peaches, and berries; yet bananas cause no problems. This only proves to me that each of us is very individual as to how our bodies react to our diet choices. I do not eat fried foods, limit red meat, and use no vitamin C supplements.

I cook most all foods from fresh ingredients, steam most of it. For drinks of choice I have been able to handle chamomile tea and of course water. In my case because the city water supply is very good and comes from a mountain source my main source of drinking water.

I still think that stress is 75% of the cause of my IC symptoms. It is sad to say but I feel better since Will's death. I am still sad, yes, but my nerves and my bladder are much better.

I have written my life story for my family to know how events beyond our control can shape our lives and our health. I was thinking back to my childhood, during World War Two; I was ten years old in 1944 and went to boarding school with my sister, in a the town of Breslau, Germany. When the bombing started the children had to leave first. My Dad was an accountant and had invested in a drug store in the town of Baden, located in the west. He told us to meet him there; it never happened. We escaped the bombing by train and went to stay with our grandparents without our belongings. We were with our grandparents for a month and found out that the entire train with all our friends and teachers had been destroyed by the bombing of Dresden. I stood on the site of a mass grave in Dresden; there is sadness that is overwhelming.

During our stay with our grandmother and grandfather, my Mother, who was a very strict and strong woman along with our little sister, joined us and my father walked all the way through Czechoslovakia and met us at our grandparents' house. We heard the last gunfire of World War Two. It was 1945 and the war was over, but in thirty minutes the Russian soldiers were in my grandparents' house; they wanted to shoot my father, looted, and took the women and molested them. My Mother was spared because we hid her in a tiny room and moved a large wardrobe closet in front of the door. Once a day we brought her food. This went on for four weeks. After the Russian soldiers left the Polish soldiers came and took what was left of our possessions.

We lived under the communists for a year. In 1946 our entire family went unnoticed to the train station and went aboard a boxcar meant to transport animals because there was no other car available for us. Our purpose was to ride across the border to a refugee camp away from the communists. There was no food, no toilet, and people were dying. All we had was straw to sit and sleep on. The trip should have taken six hours; instead, it took days as we were moved from one train to another. My Mother had a pillowcase to carry oatmeal, a little pot, and some spoons, so between trains my Dad would make a fire at the train station to cook the oatmeal. For water we heated rainwater that collected in the puddles. We knew others had used the same water to wash their feet but we used it.

When we arrived at the camp there was again only straw to sleep on, but the joy was we had food, toilets, and water. Yes, there were rats and they nibbled on me. It was hard. Like the good saying, "Tough times do not last, though people can and do. After going from one crisis to another we ended up in northern part of Germany, (Ostfriesland) near Holland, with no job or food. For four years we had first a one room then a two-room dwelling with an outhouse for a toilet. In 1950 my Dad got a job as an accountant for a church in a nearby city. I wanted to go to college and had a scholarship but had to turn it down because the housing in near the school was too expensive and I did not want to take half of my Dad's income. My sense of sadness grew along with the recognition that life does not play fair.

Now you know part of my life's story. I do think my IC symptoms and intense sense of tension are combined. I do not know if any of my thoughts will help you, but I think nerves play a big role in negative health symptoms.

My irritable bowel has been giving me trouble and that is why I wonder if the two are from the same individual's sensitivity tree. I remember a gastroenterologist speaking to our IC support group and when he asked how many IC patients had irritable bowel problems almost all 30 attendees in the room hands went up. Sadly he was surprised.

Right now my heart is acting up and I had to go into the hospital to have its rhythm restored. This is the third time. The doctor told me I need surgery when I get back from Germany. Whatever your health situation the one sure thing is that life is short and is made up of memories, good and not so good, but all family and friendships are precious. Taking care of your health is the best gift you can give yourself and your loved ones.

What I think

1. Limit how many antibiotics you take. We hear about increasing number of drug resistant bacteria, but also vaginal yeast infections, thrush, and yes, skin thrush, all are because of the repetitive use of antibiotics. Make sure your physician sends your urine out for a culture to confirm that you really do have a urinary tract infection.

2. Prelief has been my standard of care for many years. I cannot take Elmiron and have found that Prelief before meals really helps.

3. My "simple" hint is when it is a hard day or a flare is building, take a warm bath with baking soda. It may be the water environment that relaxes you or that the baking soda changes the acid on your skin and washing into vagina and urethra bringing a more neutral pH or you are granting yourself a little quiet time, but it helps.

4. Think a gentle massage for relaxation. Have heard about a study that says this is the most beneficial.

5. Diet? Does it make a difference? Yes, a thousand times yes. I wrote about Prelief really being of help, but also eating steamed vegetables, staying away from spicy foods seems basic advice and for me it helped.

6. GI upset as in cramping and diarrhea. What can you do about them? I have looked into whether I had gluten sensitivity and the genetic test was somewhat positive. I enjoy travel and have found that once out of the country my IC symptoms are much less. I think it is because of more truly natural foods and home cooked meals shared with my family and friends, meaning being with uplifting people. Seeing how in different countries they live, what they eat, and daily trips to the market, fresh air, and fresh fruits and vegetables leads me to improved health.

7. Stress, tension, anxiety are all words that bring greater pelvic pain and GI problems when my husband was battling cancer. My sleep was affected and I lost ten pounds in three months. I am not a woman who has ten pounds to lose to stress, but I did. During that dark time I had to take many medications to help me relax and sleep and now I have the pills I need for my heart. Stress, five letters that I think can bring on health disasters.

8. Reach out and find a support group. It may not even be an IC one; locally there is a very active chapter of celiac support. It gives you more information and insight into how your body works. Dr. Davis says we are more than our bladders; we need to be reminded that we are usually dealing with other health and life issues; learning about our bodies always makes sense no matter what our age.

9. Look forward. I am looking forward to a train trip from Vancouver to Toronto.

10. My children have said I am coming back to the optimistic mother they knew in childhood. I am so glad to be back.

15. Jennifer, age 41
My Life

Background

I have known Jen since she was in her early twenties and the adventurous young woman who moved to the South Bay section of California. At the point when I was wishing she were our daughter, Jennifer was into horses, living on a boat, and battling acne. As time went on, we went our separate ways. When we reconnected I would have never guessed it would have been because of the pelvic pain issues of IC. This is Jennifer's insightful story.

Jennifer's Story

My name is Jennifer and this is my story. I am 41 years old. I'm married and have three wonderful sons. My biological son is 8 and my two stepsons are 16 and 19. For the last 20 years or so I've been a secretary with varying degrees of responsibility. I was laid off from my last job and I am going to school online, full time from home.

About eleven years ago, just before my IC symptoms started, I had to have a root canal done but my health insurance wasn't due to start for a month. With that, my dentist put me on a high dose of penicillin for approximately three weeks. Towards the end of the third week I had a severe reaction to the penicillin with a whole body, red, blotchy rash, and severe itching. I didn't experience any breathing problems, thank goodness. While I don't have any concrete evidence to support this, I really feel that this incident played some kind of role in the development of my IC because my pelvic pain started directly afterward.

My IC flares started approximately eleven years ago. Symptoms were severe burning, urgency, and crazy pelvic pain. My only trigger event at that time was sexual intercourse. I was fortunate enough to have Dr. Davis and his wife, Josephine, as family friends. They recognized my symptoms and I was able to get a diagnosis before I spent what others have reported as endless, fruitless doctor visits.

During my pregnancy and after my son was born, my symptoms went away. I've been told that bladders "like" pregnancy and the bladder lining gets an extra "boost" during this time. Whatever the magic was that made the IC symptoms resolve during my one pregnancy, the result was my ability to give an honest no answer to the question if I had IC.

It wasn't until my son was 6 years old that my IC symptoms returned. When the flares did come back it was with different "triggers." Sex is no longer my trigger – YEA! My triggers now are stress, coffee, sugar, and great physical exertion. The timing is usually just before my menstrual cycle begins. For example, I'm stressed so I don't sleep very well. In the morning I'm really tired so I drink a bunch of coffee with tons of flavored creamer and sugar in it. There are 3 out of 4 triggers right there.

IC pain for me comes on like a freight train. Most of the time it is enough to wake me out of a sound sleep in the middle of the night. If I wait until morning to start rescue methods, I'm down for most of the day, unable to stand, walk, or drive.

Flare symptoms for me have actually changed over the last year. Flares used to be crazy burning, urgency, and throbbing pelvic pain. Now we can add terrible smelling urine to the list. (Oh joy) At first I thought it was truly a UTI as that had never been one of my symptoms. Three flares later, all with negative tests from a "first a.m. sample" using a home urinalysis kit, I've decided it is just part of the evolution of my condition.

I have to say that denial is very powerful. Even with pictures of my cystoscopy to prove my condition, I didn't want to have a "chronic condition," so I didn't really deal with it. Meaning, I didn't make adjustments to my life or even acknowledge that I had a medical condition that needed to be addressed (other than taking Elmiron the first time around). When you are in your thirties, you not only want to be invincible, life demands that you play the invincible role.

Even with a diagnosis of IC, my G.P. would renew my prescription for antibiotics without a urine culture any time I requested it. This eliminated the need to address my condition because in 3 or 4 days with the Rx, I would begin to feel better. What I was ignoring was that I would start to feel better in 3 to 4 days without the meds. It wasn't until seven months ago that the doctor refused to renew my Rx anymore without a positive urine culture. Having no insurance made getting a culture a $100 venture each time I needed one. Talk about a huge incentive to prevent an IC flare.

Since my G.P. "cut me off," so to speak, on the antibiotic, I've had to really look at what my flare triggers are. First, I had to identify them, and then to actually make changes to my life. I've pretty much had to cut out coffee completely and instead I drink hot herbal green tea with a smidgeon of honey. I have to admit that I occasionally slip up and get a Caramel Frappuccino from Starbucks.

During a flare my diet changes dramatically. I eat Rice Chex cereal for breakfast, egg-on-toast for lunch, and plain chicken breast with brown rice for dinner. Snack consists of hummus and tortilla chips. That diet is okay for a day or two, but it definitely gets old quickly. Why is it that we crave what we can't have? During a flare, I would give my right arm for salsa and chips, dill pickles, or a whole bag of Funyuns.

Our family dynamics aren't what you'd call typical. My husband is a long-distance truck driver so he's away a lot. I can really relate to military families. My son is one of the pickiest eaters I've ever seen so he has his own diet. This all means that my diet challenges and choices rarely affect my family. My husband's mom and sister both deal with chronic health issues so he learned early on that sometimes people hurt. While we don't wear a cast or show a temperature, pain is real and it isn't always easily explained, diagnosed, or dealt with. I am truly blessed to have a husband that gives me space and encouragement when I'm sick.

One incident that really sticks out in my memory is when my husband's aunt passed away. The funeral service was several hours' drive away. I spent the entire trip up there in the back seat of the car curled up in the fetal position until the rescue pain meds (Aleve and Uristat) could kick in.

We have quite a large blended family. I actually have only one biological sibling, a brother, but I have 9 sisters – either by marriage or due to stepfamily dynamics. My knowing about pelvic pain has helped my sisters in several ways. First, I know first-hand how bad they feel when they have a UTI and I'm able to understand and empathize just how much it really hurts. Second, it has helped me to relate rescue techniques (baking soda sitz (warm) baths) and medications that help relieve symptoms (Aleve, an antihistamine, and Uristat) until their Rx can take effect.

My greatest frustration has not been with family or friends; it's been my own lack of willpower to say no to things I know aren't the best for me. It's not my family's responsibility to change their ways or eating habits for me. That's my own battle to fight with myself.

Having someone, whether it's a friend or staff from the urologist's office call, text, or email to just "check in" with me on how my body is doing really helps. It goes a long way for me to feel not so alone in this whole process, which seems very long and a certainly frustrating journey at times.

My 45 year old female cousin almost certainly has IC, but she is in the medical field and has access to antibiotics whenever she wants/needs them. So she hasn't really dealt with Elmiron or even lifestyle changes to prevent flares. Again, denial is a powerful thing.

I am allergic to milk products. For me they produce a lot of gas, (Jet-propelled is not necessarily a good thing.) Black tea irritates my bladder and causes urgency issues. My logic is to avoid those items that would aggravate my body. I feel that any adverse reaction (histamine release) anywhere in my body can't be good for my bladder. So I try to avoid those things. I used to smoke but I don't anymore and I really don't think it had any cause or effect on my IC.

This is a bit off subject, but it alludes to my sleep and rest issues. Several years ago I was diagnosed with narcolepsy, which is an extreme urge to sleep and often causes bizarre dreams and sleep paralysis. While uncontrollably falling asleep is the most common form, there are actually 6 to 8 different varieties of the disease. The form I deal with, quite frequently, is what I call "bug dreams." They started about 22 years ago when I was 19 years old. It affects me within the first hour or so that I've fallen asleep. I "dream" that a huge spider or flying thing is about to drop on me from the ceiling or dive-bomb me. I wake myself up swinging my arms and/or scrambling to get away from it. This leads my husband to say, "There's nothing there. It's not real." My response is almost always "Yes there is - it's right there!" I can see it plain as day and at the time it is very real to me. When I finally come fully awake, whatever I'm seeing fades away into thin air and I usually go right back to sleep. Sometimes I don't even remember it's happened until my husband reminds me about it the next morning. It happens more frequently when I'm stressed. I know that if I'm having more night episodes, I have to watch what I'm doing physically and what I am eating and drinking because a flare could be one misstep away.

I have suffered from anxiety since my late teens, and lack of quality sleep definitely exacerbates that as well as my IC. Many IC patients have to get up frequently during the night to void. This hasn't been a problem for me so I'm not really sure if my IC is a contributing factor to my narcolepsy. Narcolepsy, however, I feel is definitely a contributing factor to my IC.

During the "first round" of my IC experience, we had health insurance so I was able to take Elmiron, which worked wonderfully. Taking the medicine also allowed me to not have to really deal with my triggers or my lifestyle. We don't have insurance now and can't afford to pay the full cost of it. Consequently, I work on prevention and rescue methods for when a flare does come.

For me IC has been in my life for a long time with a period of rest in the middle. Yet, I'm also at the beginning of working out what sets me off and how to prevent and deal with it. It's an ongoing and evolving process.

My answers are pretty simple. No coffee, keep sugar to a minimum, and don't overdo it physically as IT WILL come back to haunt you, much sooner than later.

I want doctors to know about IC and that it is real. The pain is enough that if there were no options for relief, suicide would be a real option for me. The pain consumes everything I have during a flare. Life STOPS until the pain can be managed. I go to bed and don't get out until it's under control. At the end of my last job, I was on FMLA (Family Medical Leave Act) so that I could be off of work without any notice for up to 2 days a month. That could be one of the reasons I was "laid off" but that's another subject entirely.

As a Mom, a good day consists of getting my son off to school on time, putting in some solid study time for my online schooling, and not feeling overwhelmed by all that I have to get done in a day.

As an IC patient, a good day consists of a day with managed pain. During a flare, everything in my normal life is put aside. All concentration is put into what to put in my body to reduce pain, and what to eat and drink that won't make it worse until it subsides. A flare for me usually lasts between 5 and 12 days.

At this point in my life I'm treading water. Elmiron is not an option right now so my focus is prevention. That might actually be a good thing though because otherwise I probably wouldn't be as aware of my body and what I put in it.

What I think
1. Antihistamine – I'm not exactly sure it helps my bladder, but if histamine release is a factor in IC, then I will definitely continue to take it.

2. Uristat is my go-to rescue drug for flares. It does not require a prescription and is effective and very inexpensive compared to all other rescue drugs. It almost completely eliminates urgency, burning, and throbbing pelvic pain. Aleve also helps with throbbing pain.

3. 8 ounces of water with a tsp. of baking soda helps for immediate relief until the rescue meds can kick in. Warm baking soda sitz baths help with immediate ease of vulvar pain.

4. The one resource that has taught me the most about IC is the "University of Real Life." I am very stubborn and hard headed. I have a lot of great information at my disposal, both literary and in the form of my urology doctor and staff. However, until I live and experience something, I don't believe or want to hear it. Unfortunately, that's been true for most things in my life, not just medically speaking.

5. For increasing my fluid intake, I found a green tea/pomegranate iced tea mix. It's bland enough to not aggravate my bladder. It has no sugar, and zero calories. I drink about four 32-ounce bottles on average a day. Before I found this iced tea mix I really struggled with getting enough liquid in my body. I really dislike plain water. My husband and I have an alcoholic mixed drink a couple of times a year. There is a lot of sugar in the mixers so I have to watch my intake as to not trigger a flare.

6. My body doesn't like chocolate very much either. There's an ingredient in dark chocolate that makes my body break out in a bright red "pin prick" rash on my face, neck, and chest. I try to stay away from it for the most part, but I really do love dark chocolate (again the craving what we can't have). The times that I've slipped up and had it, the reaction has taken 30 minutes to an hour to appear and takes a day or so to clear up. I've found that Dove brand chocolate is the most reactive brand for me.

7. During a flare, I don't go out to eat. I've managed to stay away from mandatory work related meals or unbreakable social plans.

8. As a general rule, I don't exercise. I've been thinking about Zumba, but I'm nervous it might cause a flare so I haven't been brave enough to try it yet. Short trips walking the dogs around the neighborhood have worked out fine. It's a small neighborhood so I don't really overdo it. Any extreme exertion can bring on a flare. Strenuous yard work or major house cleaning can bring one on so I have to be careful there.

9. I recently went on a two-week vacation. It really wasn't the restful vacation that one would imagine. I have lots of family dynamics and a ton of stress that goes along with it. (This is why I only make the trip every other year or so) I really dislike traveling to begin with, so the combination made for a flare that lasted from 2 days before I left until about 5 days after I got home. That resulted in a grand total of a 21-day flare. No bueno.

10. My advice to someone with a new IC diagnosis would be that everyone is different. Find out what triggers you and avoid it. Reduce acid in your diet with Tums. Reduce any histamine reactions with allergy meds (Benadryl or Zyrtec). Costco has an off-brand Zyrtec-type allergy medicine. A year's supply (360 pills) is priced fewer than twenty dollars.

16. Charleen, age 27
My Experiences to Share

Background

Charleen is 27 years old. She gives her perspective of IC/BPS and how her memories, thoughts, and experiences begin to make sense in finding ways to deal with bladder caused pelvic pain. "We shall draw from the heart of suffering itself, the means of inspiration and survival" - Winston Churchill

Charleen' Story

Hearing the name Interstitial Cystitis for the first time in the ER, I thought that I would never need to remember that name. At the time, the pain was so severe I was convinced that I had a kidney stone. After ruling out a kidney stone and any kind of infection, the female doctor that was on duty in the ER that day went the extra mile for me, thank God. This was the first person that took the time to help me get an answer in several years. I had been misdiagnosed for so long. She saw the utter hopelessness and frustration in my eyes. Honestly if I left there that day without an answer I didn't know what I was going to do. I was in so much pain and nobody would help me. I would tell people my symptoms and they would stare at me as if I were over dramatic or even making things up for attention. Thankfully this doctor called my gynecologist and together they presented me with a tentative diagnosis of IC. I was referred to an urologist where I was officially diagnosed in January of 2011.

Today as I live with IC, I look back at my life and see all the countless times someone could have helped me sooner. It's been 20 months since my diagnosis, and from that day forward it's been a constant struggle to function as a normal healthy adult. My life revolves around my bladder. IC doesn't care about your plans or your hopes and dreams. My emotional capacity to handle this daily struggle of living with bladder pain is wearing thin.

My name is Charleen, and I'm 27 years old. I am the youngest of five siblings. I grew up in Southern California and have a Bachelor's Degree in Psychology. I have a fast paced career as a sales manager for a wireless company. I am a newlywed and very happily married to the most caring and attentive man on the planet. He is my best support system and sole caregiver. I truly believe that people are placed in your life at certain times for a reason. My husband and I had only been dating for a year when he proposed; two weeks later I was diagnosed with IC. I still remember the frightened look on his face when he saw me lying in a hospital bed for the first time. It hurt me more to see the sadness in his eyes than to receive the diagnosis. It was as if I saw this life I had imagined together suddenly changing and there was nothing in my power I could do to stop it.

The one thing I never want to be is a burden to anybody. Having IC makes me feel as though I'm being a constant burden to the people in my life that love me and depend on me the most. When I met my husband I never imagined that he would be my caregiver. He has been by my side since the beginning. I am truly blessed to have such a wonderful supportive husband. I know that it hurts him to see me in pain everyday. He feels alone in this also because of the same reasons I do, nobody will understand the reality of what we go through each day.

I would say that the greatest success in educating my family about IC is that I realized who really cares about me and who doesn't. I don't mean to sound harsh, but that is the reality of being sick. People that I considered to be friends were not only uninterested in what I was going through but would also make rude and insensitive remarks. A girl I considered to be a close friend at work said, "Charleen is allergic to life!" and then laughed after I had confided in her about my illness and how I had to modify my diet.

I'm thin. When people hear that I don't or can't eat and drink a lot of things, they think I have some kind of mental problem or eating disorder. In short, it's really hard to find people who will love you even when you are sick. My husband loves me unconditionally and I don't know if I can say that about anyone else. Having him being so understanding about my condition means the world to me because no one else understands and no one else cares. People put you into their pile of problems. Out of sight and out of mind is very true, and feels very cold when it's happening to you. Funny how when you get sick, people you thought would be there for you just disappear. Having IC definitely helped me prioritize my life and put the importance of certain aspects in perspective.

As I look back at my childhood starting around age 5, I can remember my mother and my sister carrying me in to the doctor for bladder infections so painful that I could not walk. I also have memories of sitting in the bathtub as a little girl crying with my Mom yelling at me from the next room to finish the cranberry juice. Now I understand how drinking cranberry juice by the bottles was only exacerbating my symptoms all those years. I continued to have chronic bladder infections throughout my adolescents and teenage years. I had my first menstrual cycle at age 11. I noticed that the bladder pain and frequency intensified around the time of my monthly cycle. My period was extremely heavy and irregular to the point where I began taking birth control pills to attempt to regulate my cycle.

The first onset of my health problems started when I was twenty years old. The pain came on suddenly one morning when I got out of bed and I dropped to the floor and fainted. When I awoke by myself I began experiencing a sharp pain in my lower left abdomen. I went to my female doctor and she told me that I must have another bladder infection, and didn't even bother to check for anything else or even do a culture of my urine. She just sent me home with a prescription for antibiotics.

Days later I ended up in the hospital, where I remained for 10 days on fluids and everyone treated me as if I was completely irrelevant. They judged me by my looks because at the time I was young and bleach blonde. The nurses kept questioning my sexual history and were trying to infer that I may have pelvic inflammatory disorder.

One incident I will never forget is when they sent a male gynecologist whom I had never met before into my room while I was asleep and I woke up while he was performing a pelvic exam. I had never felt so violated in my entire life. I refused to see that doctor again and they couldn't understand why I was being so "sensitive". They sent in a neurologist after that because they said since they couldn't find anything medically wrong with my body, they wanted to check my brain. I had never been put through anything like that hospital stay in my life. I'm glad I learned early on how much you have to defend yourself for being in pain, especially to so called medical professionals. That experience truly opened my eyes to the medical industry and how they treat young women in pain as if all of the pain is in your head and we are there merely to seek painkillers or attention.

I sought out a female gynecologic specialist. It took 2 months to get an appointment and I waited in pain. After she and I spoke for about 15 minutes she was able to determine that I had endometriosis. The only way to treat and confirm a diagnosis of endometriosis is to perform laparoscopic surgery. After the first laparoscopy, the pain went away. By the same time the following year, I went in for my 2nd laparoscopy because my symptoms had returned. Although, after going through the trauma of another surgery and missing a semester of college, the second surgery did not relieve the pain. I woke up from that surgery screaming and crying in pain. After enduring two laparoscopic procedures within one I was referred to a different specialist who administered a new experimental drug treatment called Lupron Depot. I had that drug injected into my buttocks by the nurse once a month for eight months and it put my body through a false menopause. After about a year and a half after I began the Lupron Depot treatment I began gaining pain relief from the endometriosis.

Three years went by and my health was going in a positive direction. I was in the best shape of my life and became very active in sports and exercise. The first time I felt a different kind of more intense bladder pain and urgency was the morning of iPhone 4 launch in June. I awoke at 5 a.m. and experienced what I believe to be the first of the major signs leading up to my IC diagnosis. I work in a very fast paced, high stress, intense work environment. Looking back, this was my first flare. In addition to that I had been drinking several energy drinks a day and drinking cranberry juice by the bottles because I thought I was getting reoccurring infections. Food in combination with stress is a guarantee for an angry bladder.

After learning my limitations with IC I now know that I can't push myself as hard as I used to. I can't work standing on my feet 50-60 hours a week anymore. Since my IC diagnosis, I had been missing a considerable amount of work due to my bladder pain. I was officially diagnosed in January of 2011. I had a cystoscopy with hydrodistention in May to take pictures of the inside of my bladder. I had been in and out of work using FMLA for the majority of that year. Several months after the procedure, I was feeling intense pain in my kidneys and experiencing nausea and vomiting. The Elmiron was causing massive gastrointestinal upset and I was absolutely miserable. After getting an ultrasound, they discovered that I had several kidney stones and they needed to be removed right away due to their size. I had an extracorporeal shock wave lithotripsy (ESWL) procedure done to break up the stones. What they thought were only four stones, two in each kidney turned out to be five in the right and three in the left. At that point in my life I was in so much pain that I didn't think I would survive it. However, being the workaholic that I am I didn't take much time off work and when I returned from that surgery I went in full blast career mode and got a promotion. Little did I know, things were not getting better, they would only get worse from there. Even after I had pin pointed my bladder problem and removed the kidney stones, I still remained feeling awful everyday. I was still in pain and still missing a considerable amount of work due to my health issues. My new direct supervisor suggested I take a leave of absence so that I wouldn't cause any more instability in my performance and goals. Professionally I manage a team of 30 people. She advised me that I needed to take care of myself before I can take care of others. As harsh as it sounded at the time, I'm thankful that at least someone I work for had the compassion to see that I was genuinely struggling to physically make it through each day and needed help. Often stress from work would be the largest contributor to my bladder flares and the most frequent offender.

A flare for me is characterized by increase in frequency especially during sleeping hours. On an average day with a bladder flare I void anywhere between 2-8 times per night and between 15 to 25 times in waking hours. A flare will come with bladder spasms that create that urge to void often, abdominal pain and bloating, lower back and kidney pain, and pain that radiates down through the groin and down my legs.

Not being able to participate in life due to the challenges of IC has caused a significant strain on my success at work and in my social relationships with my friends and family as well. I have been forced to stop working because of the daily effects of IC. The majority of my time now is spent resting. Most of the time I end up canceling plans and it is difficult for people to understand why because I don't look sick. Traveling can be extremely scary and difficult also. Not knowing if I will have access to a bathroom gives me anxiety and pushes me towards staying at home. Some days the pain and urgency is so intense that a twenty-minute car ride would have me in extreme pain for several days. Also, others doubt your honesty, or question the relevancy of the condition. In reality if anybody lived but one day with IC they would understand, although I would not wish this for anybody. The most difficult message to get across to my family and friends is that I'm not going to get better, that this will never go away. Nobody understands why I can't eat and drink certain things. Most importantly, is that this is real and not something I'm making up in my head. Lastly, I want people to please stop asking me if I'm feeling better. I either have to lie every time to be polite, or if I tell people how I'm really feeling they treat me like a sick girl who has issues. I miss being normal. I miss not having to take medicine every day. I miss the days when I could be strong and independent. Now each day is spent in pain, or in anticipation for my next flare, avoiding all the things I love to do and love to eat and drink because I have IC.

Diet has played an important role in managing the symptoms of my IC. Practically everything I was consuming prior to my diagnosis was on the avoid list. Foods that I have identified to cause either a bladder flare or discomfort are the following: Potatoes are high in potassium, aspartame sweetener, sauces and dressings of all kinds all have vinegar in them, chocolate, caffeine, alcohol, coffee, tea, soda, fruit juice, cow's milk, vegetables high in oxalate like celery, processed lunch meat, brown rice, avocado, bananas, soup broths, and avoid anything processed, frozen and prepackaged. I have checked for a gluten allergy and I am not allergic to gluten, although I did eliminate eating bread for 3 months. The elimination diet was helpful because you take away all the potentially harmful foods and then you add one food back into your diet at a time so that you can see which foods are causing you discomfort.

I have found that the following foods are bladder friendly: breakfast: shredded wheat with soymilk, scrambled egg whites and fresh white bakery bread with butter. Daytime meals that are friendly are as follows: whole grain pasta with extra virgin olive oil and make a light garlic and herb sauce, steamed jasmine rice and grilled chicken breast with steamed or raw vegetables or a salad with no dressing. For deserts: a natural vanilla ice cream like Brier's can be soothing to a hot IC bladder flare and I can have an occasional sprite or 7-up to relieve my nausea and the small amount of citric acid helps to combat any more kidney stones from forming. Number one most important ingredient is water. Not just any water though. Best brand by far is Evian as it lists the mineral content on the bottle and is the most naturally pH balanced water available. When Evian is not available I look for Fiji, Smart Water and Arrowhead. Avoid water brands like Dasani and Aquafina that are simply like drinking tap water with minerals removed. What is vital to understand is that our body is the most sacred vessel we have and we must be mindful and aware of everything you are putting into your body. On average I consume 2-3 liters of water a day and my urine still looks like a carbonated cocktail.

In addition to eating the right foods you must also account for staying on a consistent regimen for exercise and make sure to take your medicines regularly to avoid pain and urgency. The medication that I have taken for IC is called Elmiron. The drug is quite expensive, made me extremely sick when I began taking it; my hair falls out by the hand full and is severely thinning on the crown and one side of my head. After taking it for 20 months I still have the same bladder pain and issues that I did when I started taking it. Only about 2% of the medication actually gets to your bladder when taken orally. I am now at the point where I am considering using a catheter to install the Elmiron medicine directly into my bladder because my symptoms are not changing. I have also been on a narcotic painkiller for 20 months called Nucynta. It is a synthetic opioid that is said to be non-habit forming. Although I do not find it to be habit forming, I have grown a tolerance for it and have had to increase my dosage over time. Pyridium is another medication that I take consistently and it does relieve the bladder spasms and helps with the urethra pain while voiding.

I have been very thankful to have the opportunity to seek physical therapy. I'm currently working with a physical therapist that specializes in urinary and pelvic floor dysfunction and pain. We have been utilizing biofeedback therapy to learn how to relax my pelvic floor muscles. I have also had one treatment of transcutaneous electrical nerve stimulation. This method was successful in relieving my pelvic pain for about 48 hours.

Sometimes it's difficult to find the silver lining in all these misfortunes. Meeting people that are compassionate makes the biggest difference in gaining a hopeful outlook on this situation. Nothing is worse than being in pain and feeling like you are all alone. Finding the right people to go to for support can be difficult. The most important thing is to remain positive and surround yourself by people that love you. I've just been diagnosed with Fibromyalgia. Now, more than ever, I'm mourning the loss of the life that I used to have and the person I was able to be. Life has somehow been put into perspective very quickly for me. All I can do at this point is try to stay positive and remain focused on healing. Yesterday is gone and tomorrow is a mystery. Everyday is a new day and the one and only thing I can control is my attitude. I can choose to be happy or I can choose to sit alone and cry. Either way, I have IC, but it doesn't have me.

What I Think

1. Some advice that I can provide for any one else out there that is struggling to control all the pain and heartache that comes along with having IC is to be positive. Even if that means that you have to remove the negative aspects of your life. If the people you are talking to for support don't care, then save yourself a tremendous deal of time and energy and cut those unsupportive people out of your life and surround yourself by people who care about you.

2. Another aspect that can be extremely helpful is reducing your stress level. If you have a stressful job, find a new one. Stress alone is the biggest culprit of IC bladder flares. Keep cortisol levels low by relaxing, meditating, stretching and doing light yoga. Listening to peaceful music can help calm the body and quiet the mind especially if insomnia or sleep disorders are present.

3. Getting regular exercise is extremely important to your overall health. I know that most of the time having IC, getting in a work out is so difficult because of the constant pain and lack of energy. At least 30 minutes of physical activity per day can help increase flexibility and reduce stress, not to mention the benefits of keeping your muscles strong and it actually combats fatigue.

4. Drink plenty of good quality bottled water and take your medications regularly, and maintain a healthy organic diet. The only beverage that is totally safe is good spring quality bottled water, so remember that when reaching for a soda or tea, it's not worth it!

5. Avoid fast food and processed foods and stick to fresh organic vegetables and fruits with lean organic free-range protein.

6. Listen to your body, and make sure that you are reacting to your symptoms and treating your flares as quickly as possible. Knowing what at home remedies to keep on hand will save you in times of crisis.

7. Always keep your medicine with you and don't hesitate to get your urine cultured when you suspect an infection or other potential problems. Listen to your doctor and be open when they recommend a treatment and don't be afraid to ask your doctor questions that concern you.

8. There will be times that you encounter individuals in the medical field who don't know what IC is and you have to educate them on what is happening to your body. They will doubt you and be suspicious. This is your body and no one knows it better than you, so stand up for yourself and insists that you be taken seriously.

9. Educate yourself on IC and the latest research. Stay informed about new treatment options and talk with your doctor about what treatment options are right for you. Don't be afraid to ask for help, because chances are, your loved ones want to help you but just don't understand what's wrong with you and how they can help.

10. Lastly, be prepared for change. Once you have IC, how you feel from day to day is going to change drastically. Come to terms with the fact that you will have good days and bad days. The bad days teach you how to manage your IC, and the good days, well, savor them because they are few and far between. Spend time with your family and surround yourself by people that love you.

17. Ron, age 46
• I Cannot Be the Only Man with BPS/IC

My name is Ron. I am 52 years old. I am a divorced father of two adult children (a son who is 29 and a daughter who is 26). Both of my parents have passed away, and I have one sister who lives in New Mexico. I am currently unemployed, and I do not have health insurance at this time. I had been working in healthcare and have accumulated 18+ years of experience.

My IC journey began five years ago. I began to experience a dull pain in my pelvic region. I didn't think much of it at the time (I think I was just hoping it would "go away"). As the year went on, the pain was becoming more intense and my quality of life was definitely changing. In addition to the pelvic pain, I was now experiencing lower back pain as well.

I made an appointment to see my Primary Care Physician (PCP) in October. He did a prostate exam, ordered a PSA blood test (which came back 0.6 which was a great relief for me). He also prescribed a 10-day course of antibiotics to determine if I simply had an infection and Vicodin for the pain. I left there that day feeling pretty confident that the antibiotics would take care of the problem, and I would soon be feeling better.

Two weeks later, I had experienced no improvement (except from the pain medication). For the first time, I began to experience anxiety and fear that I might have something more serious going on in my body. I had always been very active and energetic, but I was now feeling worn out and stressed. I was also now having problems with my urine flow and waking up to urinate during the night.

I made another appointment to see my PCP. He did prescribe Uroxatral for my urine flow symptoms and referred me to an urologist (luckily I was still working at that time and had health insurance). Although by now my stress level was quite high, I did my best to have a positive attitude that the urologist would be able to diagnosis me correctly and hopefully bring me some much-needed relief. All I wanted was pain relief. I was desperate for it.

I saw Dr. Davis in early November. We had a long conversation about my symptoms, my lifestyle and what my PCP had done to treat my symptoms. I also gave a urine sample to rule out any bacteria in my urine, and he also performed a prostate exam. He told me it sounded like I could possibly have Interstitial Cystitis (which scared the heck out of me since I had never heard of that condition). He said the only way to be sure was to undergo a procedure called cystoscopy with bladder distention. He told me I would not be awake for the procedure (which I was glad to hear) and that it is done on an outpatient basis.

My insurance company approved the procedure, and I was scheduled for late November. I must admit the morning of the procedure I was scared to death. But I kept telling myself this was a good thing, and I would have some answers finally. After the procedure, I was told that I did in fact have IC, and quite a severe case of it at that! A biopsy was also done which showed no cancer, a HUGE relief. I was given some photos of my bladder lining. My bladder lining looked like red meat; I had never seen anything so awful in my life!

Before I was released to go home, I met with a dietician to go over what would now become my "new diet". I was shocked to hear about all the foods I would need to avoid. Basically, acid was the enemy, and I had no idea so many foods were considered "acidic." I was also prescribed Elmiron, and a medication to help with the burning I would experience over the next few days. As I left the hospital to go home I realized my life had just changed forever. The first 24 to 36 hours after the procedure were awful. But I somehow managed to get through it.

The diet changes were extremely difficult for me. It's really quite different than most "diets." For example, fruit is good for you right? WRONG! I had always enjoyed fruits of all kinds. Well now, the only fruits I can eat that won't affect my bladder are pears, blue berries and bananas. Vegetables for the most part seem to be okay for me. I have managed to eliminate soda, alcohol, tomato products and chocolate. I can occasionally get away with drinking a cola or a few beers at a party. But those are rare occasions, and I am fully aware that I may trigger a "flare." I have gotten pretty good now at detecting a possible "flare." An excellent example is recently I was grocery shopping, and I spotted a jug of green tea with ginseng on sale and bought it since all I drink is bottled water. The morning after drinking a glass I woke up with bladder pain. Well with some simple experimenting, I can now cross green tea off of my list of things I can drink.

Even with the diet changes and taking Elmiron, I was still always in what I'll call "general pain." I never had a pain free day. In fact, most days were still affecting my quality of life. I tried every over the counter pain medication I could find. I tried baking soda in a glass of water, which did offer some very minimal and short lasting relief. I tried a product called Prelief, which is supposed to remove acid from the food you eat.

My PCP would continue to prescribe Vicodin, which I used only as directed, but I knew I could not live the rest of my life taking that medication. But it was the only thing that allowed me to function on a fairly "normal basis."

I was laid-off from my job in three years ago because the company was going to close. I wasn't even offered Cobra insurance! I was told that since the company was basically declaring bankruptcy, they weren't required to offer it. Now I had additional stress because any physician visits or prescriptions would have to be paid "out of pocket." I did receive unemployment, but it was only about half of what I was making. I was now doing my best to look for work and manage my IC pain. The pain medication I was taking was becoming less affective. I did not get much quality rest. I was slipping into a very dark place. I felt alone, discouraged and angry. Pain brings out the worst in people; I felt like "giving up."

My quality of life was now at a new low. I became not much fun to be around. I had to constantly cancel plans with friends and family because I was so exhausted. Why did I have to be in the approximate 1% of males who develop this disease? What did I do to deserve this? Luckily for me my girlfriend had been extremely supportive through all of this, but I began to fear I might lose her eventually. I mean how can I expect her to hang in there indefinitely, knowing there was no cure for IC?

In June, two years ago I had an appointment with my PCP. I didn't realize it, but that appointment would turn out to be the beginning of the road back to a much better quality of life. He informed me that he was no longer comfortable prescribing Vicodin for my bladder and back pain. At first I was devastated. But I have read that physicians are very careful when it comes to prescribing narcotic pain medication.

Even though I had been taking it as prescribed, there was still a potential for addiction, not to mention the possible long term affects it may have on my liver. I was instructed to see Dr. Davis regarding my pain issues.

I saw Dr. Davis in July the following year. I explained that my PCP would no longer prescribe pain medication for me. He was glad because he doesn't believe in treating chronic pain with narcotics. He gave me a prescription for what he called "an oldie but a goody" drug called amitriptyline. I was to take one (1) tablet every night 2 hours before bedtime. He also gave me another prescription for Elmiron since I qualified to receive it for free. It didn't work for me 3 years ago, but it wouldn't hurt to try it again.

I was lucky that I didn't have any withdraw symptoms when I stopped taking Vicodin. I had read horror stories about that, but since I took them as prescribed, I suppose that made a difference. But I was of course in severe pain without it. The amitriptyline seemed to be working to some degree. I slept better and I didn't have that raging pain in my bladder when I woke up. I was a bit "groggy" though (kind of like a hangover). But I was more than willing to feel that way rather than be in severe pain! I started to feel that maybe, just maybe, this time we had found a medication that would work. Of course I still had to stay on a very strict diet. I needed to keep my stress level down as it had proved time after time to be a trigger for increased pain. I continued with this "plan" for about a year. I had bad days when my pain level was very high. I know it was because of the stress of being unemployed along with juggling my bills. I have been blessed to have always had a job, and it was incredible to me how hard it was to find work!

By May, the amitriptyline began to lose its effectiveness, and I began having more bad days than good days. I became very discouraged and frustrated. I was back to spending many days alone at home, unable to participate in activities with friends and family. I was becoming that cranky guy again. What had become mended relationships were again becoming strained. It was difficult for my girlfriend to spend time with me because I had become so angry. I was close to ending our relationship for "her sake" because I couldn't stand the person I had become. They say sometimes you have to hit rock bottom before you can rise up. I was definitely at that place.

The pain had such a hold on me at this point. I made another appointment to see the urologist in a month. I must admit I didn't have a lot of hope as I drove to my appointment. I really felt completely helpless and almost like a prisoner to IC. As it turns out I met with the Physician Assistant (PA) that day. I explained my situation to her as simply as I could. She prescribed a relatively new pain medication called Nucynta to be taken every 6-8 hours as needed. She prescribed the lowest dose (50mg). Apparently this medication was "narcotic like" but with less chance of addiction and less potential constipation which a lot of narcotics can cause. She also prescribed Allegra 60mg (an antihistamine) to be taken twice a day. I did not meet with the urologist that day, but was instructed to come back the following month for a follow-up visit. So off I went with as much of a positive attitude that I could convince myself to have.

After filling the prescriptions I went home and took an Allegra and a Nucynta tablet. I had a morning appointment so I was able to take a second Allegra before bed as well as another Nucynta. For the first time in nearly 4 years, I woke up the next day PAIN FREE!! I couldn't believe it. It truly did feel like a miracle. I didn't know how to act or what to think. I did have some minor pain later that day. But I took a Nucynta tablet and the pain was completely gone in less than an hour! I called my girlfriend and my kids to share the good news. I was almost in tears when I shared the news with them. For the first time in years, I had real hope!

For the time leading up to my next appointment I continued taking the Allegra twice a day. I only took the Nucynta when I needed it and I never needed more than 2 tablets a day to keep my pain level at "0". I was sleeping better, and my mood was great. I went back to bowling. My relationship with my girlfriend has never been better, and my kids are very happy to have their Dad "back." I could not wait for my next appointment with Dr. Davis so I could share my good news!

I know I must remain cautiously optimistic. I know there's a chance that maybe the medications will someday lose their effectiveness. But I believe attitude is everything, and I'm choosing to enjoy this new "freedom", live my life and be thankful that through a lot of trial and error, I finally have the formula that gives me the best chance to live a normal life. As I write this, I'm happy to report that I have a pain level of "0!"

This is what I'd like those who are suffering as I once did to know.

What I Think:

1. See an urologist as soon as possible if you think you may have IC.

2. Educate yourself about the condition, but try not to over-analyze.

3. Remember it may get worse before it gets better; patience is a virtue.

4. Strictly follow an IC diet & learn to recognize YOUR "triggers."

5. Keep a diary of everything you eat. You won't always have to do this but at the beginning of your journey; it is a very useful tool.

6. Learn to control and minimize STRESS. The less stress in your life the better.

7. Learn to advocate for yourself. We do not have to live with high level of pain. You CAN improve your quality of life.

8. Get as much rest as you can. You will be more prepared to function in your daily activities.

9. Never, ever give up! If you work with your Urologist you can no doubt find the best plan of attack. Remember, patience will pay off. It took nearly four years for me to get my IC under control. Had I acted sooner rather than later to address my symptoms, I may not have had to suffer so long.

10. If you're not happy with your current urologist, get a second opinion. The condition is still a bit of a mystery, and perhaps a different perspective may bring better results

When you're feeling up to it, get out and enjoy the world. You deserve it!

18. Jan, age 57
Email Conversations: Working on BPS/IC Recovery

Background

As a wife, mother of two children, teacher, soccer player, and runner, Jan has a full-time life. Her IC symptoms became very evident at the age of 57. She reached out to the Citrus Valley IC Support Group through www.icaction.com for help. These email exchanges with Jo illustrates Jan's journey back to a civilized bladder that was accomplished with a focus toward healing and finding the support that helped her take charge.

The following communication spans more than a year as Jan and Jo learn from each other. The person-to-person communication via email shows that support can come from many sources, and two people can make a support group.

Jan shares her ability to understand how a stable health situation can turn on choices that we make everyday.

As you read the following email exchanges of Jan's path to understanding her body's reactions and dealing with BPS/IC is an ongoing process. We hope you will find a clearer direction for your own heath solutions.

FEBRUARY

From: Jan
To: support@icaction.com
Sent: Fri, Feb 22 at 4:00 PM
Re: Contact from ICaction.com

I read Lisa's story and was encouraged. I have just been diagnosed and am looking for information to help myself. I would like to know how she took action when she had a flare, and what meds her doctor prescribes. So far, my doctor has only told me to avoid coffee, tea, chocolate, citric, and alcohol, and gave me Detrol LA to take as needed. There is no local support group in my area, and my doctor has given me little to go on. What I read online is very scary in terms of long term

Thank you for being there.

Jan

From: support@icaction.com

To: **Jan**
Sent: **Saturday Feb 23, at 6:18 PM**
Re: **Contact from ICaction.com**

Jan:

This will be a long email.

I am Jo Davis and work for Citrus Valley Urology in Glendora, CA. I work with Lisa and will share your email with her.

We have IC clinic every Tuesday. As you read on our web site, we also have a Support Group since 2001.

You did not say how long you have had the level of bladder or urinary symptoms that resulted in seeking medical attention. Most have urinary urgency, frequency, and then pelvic pain hits. This can take years before you seek help.

In fact, many of our support group members and patients remember being the one who had to go to the bathroom more than other family members or friends since they were children, or they report that their mom or a close relative shared the same experiences.

BPS/IC (Interstitial Cystitis) appears to have more than a possible inherited component. Add daily stress, food, and drink intake of our US diets, and reproductive hormones functions, (many report pain increases 7 to 10 days before a period.) IC is more common than is reported or treated. You did not say your age, but in our office the average age that looks for medical help is 35. So we are talking about tending to significant others of all categories from boyfriends to spouses, to children, to relatives, home, school, and work demands. And who in this world has time for any physical problem? Our bodies may have been telling you for years that something wasn't right, but most of us step right over the signals.

The best part of your email is you know what you have to work on - hardest part - caring for yourself.

Though you said the medication and information shared by your physician was limited, please know that if he recognized IC, that is a great leap forward. It put you on the road to understanding how to deal with IC symptoms and begin the healing process.

Background

IC is very prevalent, but because there is no urine test or blood test or any other way to determine IC other than a bladder exam, and that may or may not alert a physician to IC. As a general observation, the medical profession either rejects the diagnosis and/or pretends it does not exist or treats it with minimal time investment; unfortunately there are still a rare group of physicians who work with IC patients to help them begin to take the measures to help heal their bladder linings, control the symptoms, and regain control of their lives.

IC is a medical condition that, to work on repair, takes time to set up an individual plan and time to heal. This is not a quick-fix problem because time has gone by and symptoms were tolerated or not diagnosed and the bladder lining continued to be damaged, and bladder nerves go on constant alert. Also because IC symptoms often present themselves as bladder infection symptoms and a simple clean catch office donated urine specimen shows white cells, or red cells - antibiotics are often incorrectly prescribed. IC appears to be sensitivity, inflammation response – not an inflammation caused by infection.

The zinger is that because of the breaks or thinning of the bladder lining, IC patients are more vulnerable to bladder infections. Lesson learned is that the MD office should send the urine specimen to a laboratory for culture to find out if there is an infection. If there is infected urine the sensitivity part of the lab procedure will list what medication is the proper one to be prescribed; this is a vital part of health care that is too often stepped-over with an antibiotic prescription as the only step taken.

IC is recognized as an inflammatory response of the cells of our bladder linings.

The prevailing opinion is that IC happens because bladder cells that produce the protective mucus that protects the bladder wall, muscles, nerve and nerves from the caustic chemical in urine do not regenerate as quickly as they need to.

Urine is mostly potassium and other rejected substance as dyes and preservatives, all caustic, but for a normal bladder lining this is usually not the problem. The thick mucus cover (GAG) layer protects the bladder wall with its millions of nerve endings and muscle fibers; with IC the bladder lining is not well protected.

Much like a sun burn that has salt put on it, or the inside of your mouth if you have an ulcer after taking a sip of a hot drink – you know quickly that you have reinjured your self. So you protect the area and cool it down until the cells are renewed and the injured area is healed.

With IC the cells struggle to regenerate. And when we do not know what is going on, we keep re-injuring ourselves.

There are two phases to the repair process: (1) Protecting the bladder with medication and a diet that stays away from what your physician suggestions, the stimulants like coffee, tea, chocolate and add no spices (they are acids) or MSG (monosodium glutamate) additives. MSG unfortunately is in so much of our packaged and processed foods including canned soups. This is what makes the very food and liquids we drink cause inflammatory responses.

Though organic foods cost a bit more, going "true" organic is what we advise rather than limiting your fruits and vegetables. (2) Symptom control - Diet as well as medications, such as Detrol LA, while healing, that reduces the resting pressure in the bladder muscles fibers that have not been sufficiently protected by the GAG layer.

Suggestions

Step 1.

Write down what you eat and drink for 3 days. *Change Nothing.*

Why? To see what your eating pattern really is. You may find that you go for long periods with no food intake. This is easily solved with a packet of almonds to keep the stomach acid down. If your stomach and intestines are happy your bladder has a fighting chance.

Also write down from 0 to 10 the pelvic pain you are having. 1, 2, 3, level of discomfort, we are usually able to go on with life's demands. At a pain level of 4 and above it gets much more difficult to deal with daily living. And how many times during a 24-hour day do you void? 8 to 10 is the "normal" for a 24-hour period. This number of voids means we have taken in the amount of fluids our body needs.

Is there a symptoms pattern, i.e. long periods of sitting and perhaps ignoring that you should urinate but wait instead? Note how many times during the night do you get up to void when you should be sleeping. If it is more than once this makes a huge impact on the quality of your health and life.

Drinking water that has a mineral content (spring) – not reverse osmosis, or "purified" brands as Aquafina or Dasani because these strip the minerals, and it increases the acid content. For people struggling with IC, a small increase in acid content makes a big difference. Drink more water – yes, you will void more, but your urine will be more dilute and less caustic.

Step 2.

Medication - Elmiron (pentosan polysulfate sodium) is the only FDA-approved medication for IC. It is slow, but it works with the help of your diet choices and additional medication to control the negative symptoms until your body settles down. You did not say if your MD has prescribed this medication. The mechanism of repair is thought to be that Elmiron slowly covers the breaks and thin sections of your bladder lining with the medication and gives your body a chance to heal.

Symptom control – please discuss with your physician the use of Elavil (amitriptyline). When it is prescribed in 10 mg to 25 mg dose orally and taken about 2 hours before bedtime; it helped control the urge to void during the night if getting up to void is a problem. Also an antihistamine such as Allegra or generic fexofenadine or Claritin (both now sold without a prescription) may help because of the inflammatory aspect of IC. Benadryl (diphenhydramine) has been around for a long time; it does make most people sleepy and may be worthwhile before bedtime. Also discuss the use of an antidepressant because pain has chemically changed you. If life seems overwhelming, know that serotonin production is being compromised by your pelvic pain. Yes, this is a long list of pills. But each represents an avenue of control of IC symptoms as your body regroups.

Step 3.

Pain relief - Tylenol PM has Benadryl as its magic for nighttime rest. An antacid like Tums or as basic as baking soda; a teaspoon in a half glass of water followed by another cup water, and then using at least a cup in a warm bath helps lower temporally the acidity or pH of the urine and gives comfort and often at least temporally helps a painful episode.

Narcotics – As an example, the use the much used and abused Oxycodone, Oxycontin or generically sold under the name, hydrocodin, I can simply answer, no. IC is chronic and controllable; masking the pain by numbing your mind does not help the process of healing. If this was a broken leg, directly after surgery, or terminal painful disease as cancer, using whatever works to control pain is a valid argument because you are addressing a short term or not curable condition. I think this is about all anyone can absorb at one reading. And these are only a few suggestions.

It will take a while to understand what is going one with your body and it will take work to control. You will get better. Please keep writing us about your progress and concerns.

Dr. Davis is more than open to you physician calling and with your approval disusing any other course of treatment with him.

Thank you for reading so much.

JO

From: Jan
To: support@icaction.com
Sent: Saturday, Feb 23, at 1:04 PM
Re: Contact from ICaction.com
Jo:

I so appreciate your reply and Dr. Davis's willingness to talk to my physician.

I should have given you more information about my situation. I am 57 years old and first started noticing pain in my vulva about a year ago when I had surgery for a very deep Bartholin cyst. I had pains down my leg and other discomfort the year I was aware of the cyst, so I didn't think of any other cause. This past year, I have had several times when the labia area inside seemed inflamed but after a few days it would get better. What led me to the IC diagnosis was that I was starting to ache in my pelvic area, but without frequency or pain when urinating. I also had a small amount of blood in my urine that did not stop after antibiotics.

My gynecologist is the one I have been working with; he did a procedure to look in my urethra and said that my bladder was scarred. I heard him say to his nurse that I had signs of Interstitial Cystitis but he did not say it directly to me. He told me that my bladder was scarred, and than gave me the diet advice and the medicine I mentioned.

Since the diagnosis, I tried a cup of decaf one day and started having pressure. That lasted a couple of days and went away. I stayed away from coffee after that. I had been drinking about 3 cups of coffee a day before the diagnosis and stopped it immediately. My doctor had not mentioned alcohol, so I had one glass on Valentine's Day and really suffered with pressure and pelvic pain. That finally subsided, and I won't touch it again!

I am otherwise very healthy with an excellent blood panel and actively playing women's soccer and jogging.

My hope is to start a treatment program as soon as possible to start building up the gag layer. I have already started a basic food diet from the ICA website.

I have been online all weekend gathering information. There are several urologists in the central coast area, but I am concerned with finding the one with experience in treating this. I also need a positive attitude along with it. When I asked my gynecologist if it would get worse, he looked tense and said it wouldn't kill me, but I wished he had recommended I see an urologist the day he diagnosed me.

I am so grateful to you for replying with so much information and suggestions. I also like your positive approach to saying that it can be repaired.

In terms of eating, I eat three meals a day and snacks in between. By the way, I thought almonds were a trigger food!

I am not on the Elmiron or any other drugs you mentioned. I hope by contacting a local urologist, that I can get that kind of support. If you can recommend one in my area, please let me know.

Thank you again, it helps to be in contact with other people. I am so sad about this, and the effect it could have on my family. I am an older mom with a 10 year old and a 14 year old, and I teach full time. I am very concerned about causing problems with my job if it keeps progressing. So my action plan is doing the diet, and finding the medical support I need as soon as possible.

Jan

From: support@icaction.com
To: Jan
Sent: Sunday, Feb 24, at 10:36 AM
Re: Contact from ICaction.com

Jan,

Thank you for the added information.

You did not say if urinary function has been compromised in any way.

Yes, vulvar pain is often a reflection of IC and not a separate problem. Anatomically there are three main nerves that emerge from the spinal column at the sacral area. They innervate each of us from the belly button down. So we can have toe pain, thigh pain, vulvar, clitoral, pain etc. all reflecting distress from the pelvic region as the bladder nerves communicate its painful message to our lower body.

Sexual intercourse is in need of lubrication for comfort and pleasure. This can be a commercial lubricant like Astroglide or virgin olive oil. The main point is to find out because basic vaginal dryness needs medication treatment.

A Thought

Ask your doctor about Valium, generically diazepam. It is a muscle relaxant and small dosage amount inserted in the vaginal canal can bring relief of pelvic spasms - nerve pain of IC - this is reflected in the vulva. Valium used as a vaginal insert was explored for the one purpose - to lessen post intercourse pain. Sounds silly, but the medication used this way has worked for many.

Ask your attending physician what he thinks about you trying this course of treatment.

Our experience at the IC Clinic began with a patient whose job demands full time walking and interacting with the public. She has had success with this medication and method of delivery. She reported it took her three weeks of staring at the bottle to give it a try, but for her it works.

There is quite a bit of information available on the web. I will forward an email with the section that discusses this topic to share with your MD.

Fact is that so much of what we have learned about IC comes from the patients and the support group.

Another avenue of healing is physical therapy that is also called pelvic massage or perineal massage – As you can guess this physical therapy is very intimate and for many a leap of faith. This method of massage is to relax the pelvic floor and release the tension in the pelvic muscle/nerves. Very specialized and as an example there is only one source for this treatment in our area; as a result we have few patients who have availed themselves of this method of treatment. With some guidance for the gynecologist perhaps a partner can learn some of the relaxation techniques. This is not for just expectant moms.

Along those lines, I have come to realize over the years that we have to treat all muscles and tendons with respect when we exercise or do any stressful activity. If you have a muscle that has been stressed for whatever reason the first thing an athlete does is ice the injured muscle to reduce the chance of swelling caused by inflammation of the injury because the swelling that comes with inflammation brings pressure on the nerve fibers.

So after you exercise, shop, sit or ride in a car for a long period, sex included, frozen gel packs really help. When frozen always wrap a frozen gel pack to protect your skin, and placed between your legs to cool the perineal area and translates to helping your urethra, vulvar, bladder inflammation to be reduced. Lisa wised me up because I was using heat and she said, "Why would you put heat on sunburn (inflammation)?" – She was right.

You did not mention low back pain, but this often is present with IC and is a reflection of muscles tensing in the back from the bladder or vulvar pain. This is when heat helps to relax the muscles that have not been injured but are tense from reflected pain.

Ice between the legs and heat lower back.

About coffee – decaffeinated coffee has reduced caffeine, and caffeine is indeed a muscle stimulant, but decaffeinated coffee continues to have an acid content.

There is low acid coffee on the market. Basically they have bathed the beans in an antacid. Not drinking such beverages is the best until you know your IC symptoms are under control.

An important piece of information you shared is the positive reaction you had to the dismissal of coffee and alcohol from your diet. You are at least to some degree diet sensitive to acidic foods.

Almonds are one of the few nuts that have a good track record for not causing a pelvic pain reaction. For those who do not like the fact that they are a bit harder to chew than some other nuts we suggest organic or home made almond butter.

Also lookup an antacid product - "Prelief" – over the counter – it targets the acid in food. Many IC Clinic and Support Group swear by it. If acid is the main trigger it will be of value.

We have several patients who have taken the dietary route alone, but most combine both diet and medication as a way to stabilize the bladder symptoms. My concern is the degree of pain you are experiencing and your teaching duties may require medication to help calm the pelvic and/or vulvar pain.

Your gynecologist can prescribe all medication - you do not have to see an urologist.

Please do ask about Elmiron. If he stops there with medication, an urologist would be a good resource for specialized care. However, you are correct, an urologist in general will give more guidance that what you have now. I will ask Tuesday at work what, if any, resources are in your area. Sometimes the ICA network lists MD/urologists contacts. Also the Elmiron website can be helpful for physician contacts.

As another note: At 57 years of age, hormones are a great influence in health issues. Did your gynecologist address vaginal tissue and the urethral need for estrogen? Estrace cream, small amount topically applied to the vagina and urethra can be a great help.

Swear my emails are not usually this long. Hope this is helping. JO

From: Jan
To: support@icaction.com
Sent: Sunday, Feb 24, at 2:28 PM
Re: Contact from ICaction.com

Jo:

Thank you so so much for your reply again. It helps to not feel entirely alone on this.

My husband is coming back from a skiing trip for the weekend, and I have to let him know what is happening. I feel very sad about this.

I am grateful you mentioned Prelief. Since this last flare up that started last Thursday, I have been feeling irritated in my bladder area; like someone scrubbed it with a scrub brush. I am eating the healthy diet, but can only find relief for a while when I take some baking soda in water. I have had urgency feelings since last Thursday, but it is not clearing up like it has in the past. I can see that my symptoms are progressing.

I am hopeful you can find someone in this area on Tuesday when you check. Otherwise I will check with the gynecologist. I do not know if he will be willing to work with me.

I am hoping to start the medicines as soon as possible to help maintain and rebuild on what I have before I do more damage. The Valium might be helpful to help me with work. I will see how it goes this next week. I am concerned about urgency, but I do have a kindergarten teacher next door with a bathroom available. I am going to tell her about my situation so if she sees me going often she can check on my class if needed.

Jan

From: Jan
To: **support@icaction.com**
Sent: **Monday, Feb 25, at 6:31:04 PM**
Re: **Contact from ICaction.com**

Jo,

Thank you again for the long email. I would be so uninformed and depressed if I hadn't made contact with you. I am so grateful for all the information you are sharing. Your news is action oriented and very helpful to me.

I am just starting out on this journey and there is so much to absorb. When I look at the IC website, I never know if I am going to read something helpful or some that will scare me. By the way, I told my husband and shared your first email with him that has the background on it. I don't think he realized how serious it can be, but was impressed by the possibilities you shared. He is very supportive.

I have been doing better with the pain by taking a few Tums. I was able to line up some Prelief in my area at Wal-Mart. They don't usually carry it but ordered it right away at a discount I hope. I will pick it up tomorrow and try it.

I am relieved that the pain in my vulva has diminished. I have noticed yesterday and today that when I sit for a while, I start to ache in my pelvic area. If I get up and walk around, it helps. I hope being on my feet as a teacher will help. I did take one of the Detrol LA this morning to help.

I am curious if your clinic has anything on an alkaline diet. I really miss my daily dose of peanut butter.

As far as my gynecologist, I am on the Estring (estrogen) for vaginal dryness, but he has mentioned nothing about urethral tissue.

I will keep the Valium in mind if things get worse.

I am hoping your clinic will be able to help me connect with someone in this area when you check on Tuesday. I am hopeful I can find someone who can be encouraging and positive, and give me the optimal treatment.

Thank you again for being so helpful.

Jan

From: support@icaction.com
To: Jan
Sent: Tuesday, Feb 26, at 12:34 PM
Re: Contact from ICaction.com

Jan:

Let me introduce you to Joan. She works with me as a patient advocate in our IC Clinic. Joan has been on Elmiron, is not sensitive to iodine, and has had the symptoms of Vulvodynia beginning 15 years ago and now has no symptoms if she stays on this fairly simple regimen. She has gone back to a regular diet with no coffee or tea and watches the acid food intake and watches for artificial coloring and preservatives. She is big on no MSG (monosodium glutamate.)

Joan takes Elmiron.

Her suggestions begin with:

1. National Vulvodynia Association (hrrp://www.nva.org/)
2. Low oxalate diet - example beans are high, green peppers, - not IC but specialized
3. Add calcium citrate to you diet – one brand is Citracal with only D.
4. Notes: Citracal is made up of calcium citrate and not carbonate – calcium citrate is more easily absorbed than calcium carbonate.
5. Aveeno (oatmeal) treatment as a soak or compress to the vulva before bedtime or after intercourse.
6. Lidocaine cream or ointment – we discussed but she suggested the prescription form that is the ointment and is 5%. Over the counter lidocaine is cream and is 4%.
7. Also an antihistamine
8. Definitely Estrace cream
9. Vitamin E capsules – puncture and use contents as a balm for an irritated perineal area.

Joan just reviewed a book titled "Because You Care" – It is a great one for your husband to read or you read selections to him.

You can order it from the ICA at www.icahelp.org.

Jo

From: Jan
To: support@icaction.com
Sent: Tuesday, Feb 27, at 1:26 AM
Re: Contact from ICaction.com

Thank you very much for the info from Joan. I appreciate it and had never heard of that condition.

My main question right now is if your clinic has any knowledge of a doctor to work with me in the Central Coast area.

Please let me know.

Thank you,

Jan

From: support@icaction.com
To: Jan
Sent: Tuesday, Feb 27, at 5:58 PM
Re: Central Coast an IC MD

Jan:

Can you give me your zip code and the number of miles you are able to travel for the appointments?

Thank you, Jo

From: Jan
To: support@icaction.com
Sent: Tuesday, Feb 27, at 1:26 AM
Re: Contact from ICaction.com

I was glad to hear from you.

In terms of miles, that is hard to say. I am getting achy after my twenty five mile commute to work, but my urgency has gotten back to normal. I guess I could use ice packs for the achiness.

So the miles could be 0 to 90 miles.

I am considering coming down to your clinic to get started with a treatment plan. I know you offered to have Dr. Davis work with an urologist in this area. Please advise…

Thank you for your help again. The ice on the front and the heat on the back pain treatment you mentioned are very helpful. I was able to order the Prelief through Wal-Mart. So at least I have some tools right now.

Jan

From: support@icaction.com
To: Jan
Sent: Wednesday, Feb 28, at 6:03 AM
Re: Central Coast an IC MD

Here is one contact. Located in Encino and that might be a bit of a stretch for you. But it is a place to start. Also note practice is an association of urologists. So ask if any of the MDs have an interest in IC. Hope this helps.

Jo

From: Jan
To: support@icaction.com
Sent: Thursday, Feb 29, at 7:55 AM
Re: Contact from ICaction.com

Jo:

Thank you for the info you have been sending on the doctors. The closest one you mentioned is about 60 miles away. I did contact the local urology association you mentioned and they recommended a Dr. C. to me who they say is the best in the area. I have set up an appointment for March 14.

I will also keep in mind that you suggested that Dr. Davis would be willing to consult with a local doctor in my treatment.

Do you have more information on the elimination diet? I was surprised when I to tried drinking some carrot juice and it resulted in urgency.

Thank you so much for all your information and support.

Jan

From: support@icaction.com
To: Jan
Sent: Thursday, Feb 29, at 12:57 PM
Re: Physicians, etc.

Jan:

Our office takes most insurance plans, and a quick call to the office will confirm that yours is fine. My concern is one of distance and continuity of care. Dr. Davis has often spoken to urologists around the country as they work on a care plan and that route may be the best if Dr. C. is open to the suggestion.

There is care oversight that needs to be easily available at the beginning of your recovery so my advice is to go through with the March 14th appointment and make the determination whether you have to go further in you search or miles traveled to find medical care.

Other thoughts:

1. To focus quickly on your care, call ahead and have Dr. C's office request a copy of your records from the gynecologist

and/or other physician you have seen in the past year. Then the information will be there on the 14th.

2. You will have to sign a release so they can request your records and that can be done by fax. You can request a copy of the information, but most offices charge for the service, but do not charge if it's MD to MD.

3. Your medical records belong to you. Physicians are only caretakers of your records. A three ring binder and some plastic sleeves and you will have a record of your medical care that you can take with you wherever you go. Old fashioned but works.

4. After you visit with Dr. C. have their office make a copy for you of your visit records.

5. Before the MD visit make a list of all the surgeries you have had since birth, all medical needs to visit a physician in the past two years, and all medications you take – make two columns – prescribed and over the counter, vitamins included. This will help you fill out the forms that always come with a first visit and should be part of your binder info.

6. You need to keep a record of your MD visits and procedures. Ask the urologist if he has the O'Leary/Sant and the Parson's Pain (PUF) questionnaires. These are good for keeping a record of your bladder improvements given there is no urine or blood test for IC. The questionnaires put numbers to the changes in your health and track changes.

Reading suggestions and reference guides:

Interstitial Cystitis Survival Guide
Robert M. Moldwin, MD, FACS
A good general knowledge book/primer. The great news is we are beyond "survival" in dealing with IC.

Confident Choices
Julie Beyer, RD
She is a Registered Dietitian, has IC, and took that knowledge she has gained and mixed it with other source information, recipes, and tracking forms

A Taste of the Good Life
Bev Lauman
First book that linked a personal look at diet and recipes

MARCH

From: Jan
To: support@icaction.com
Sent: Sunday, Mar 2, at 6:44 AM
Re: Contact from ICaction.com

Jo,

Do you have any suggestions for the pelvic pain? I have been waking up in the middle of the night for the last week with aching in my pelvic area. It has really starting to affect my sleep. I eventually go back to sleep but it is difficult.

I have tried the Tylenol before I go to sleep but it hasn't seemed to help. After taking one last night at 9 p.m., I still woke up about 2 a.m.

Jan

From: support@icaction.com
To: Jan
Sent: Sunday, Mar 2, at 10:29:24 AM
Re: Physicians, etc.

Jan:

If you are addressing what is called a "flare" - this would mean that your pain level has increased. It can happen suddenly or begin to creep up to a greater degree than you have experienced as a constant.

Sleep time is precious and self-rescues may be of value.

Self-rescues are based on a combination of items.

1. As mentioned before - good old fashion baking soda. A cup of baking soda or more in warm bathwater followed by a spa soaking helps reduce the acid in the perineal area. Also, I think, helps your body and mind take a deep breath. This I would try as a bedtime decompression time.

2. Baking soda - a teaspoon in ½ cup of water - chug it and then follow with regular water, you will burp. This is about 2 hours before bedtime. Helps reduce the acid content of your urine for a short time and that is often enough to calm the bladder down for a good nights sleep. There is a warning on the baking soda package about extended

use if you have high blood pressure. But one or two times will not affect hypertension.

3. You indicated Tylenol, but was it Tylenol PM - the one that has the Benadryl? I wrote about a nonprescription Benadryl that can be taken about 2 hours before bedtime.

Sleep and the antihistamine effect helps.

4. Call it concern, call it tension, call it stress, all can push the pain level up.

5. Ice pack wrapped in a towel - perineal area at bedtime also helps - And a warm area around the lower back. Both work to put a person to a deeper sleep and have a less likely chance of awaking. Or if awakened with these two different elements falling back to sleep can be easier.

6. Over the counter – non-prescription antihistamines such as Claritin, Allegra - Do not make you sleepy but given the green growth outside my windows, seasonal allergies may also be playing a part in a flare and or a sleepless night.

JO

From: Jan
To: support@icaction.com
Sent: Monday, Mar 3, at 6:30 AM
Re: Physicians, etc.

Jo,

I tried the warm bath and slept more soundly. But the pain is still there.

Jan

From: support@icaction.com
To: Jan
Sent: Thursday, Mar 6, at 10:43 AM
Re: Physicians, etc.

Jan:

Glad that there are some rescues that can help you at least a little with sleep. One woman said to me that it was too bad she could not live her life in a baking soda bath. It would be so much easier.

Would you describe what you have experienced as an increase in pelvic pain from what you have previously experienced? Is the increase in intensity and/or location of the pelvic pain more than you have experienced the past? Is this a prolonged flare? Flare, meaning more distress in urinary symptoms jumps up. If the source can be identified more often than not it is after sexual intercourse, eating or drinking something that is off the OK chart. Spring allergy time, stress of life going through an over whelming passage – as preparing for a trip even a fun one, doing taxes, and/or work demands.

And on top of it all – pain feeds on itself as the adrenalin flows.

Rescues are important in taking charge and help our bodies settle down. But self-help rescues can go only so far in helping to stop the pelvic pain. The point is to decide when this is a situation you can handle and when the symptoms are running away from your ability to quiet or control them.

You can see that some causes can be medicated but others cannot. My opinion is that, at this point, you probably need to be on additional medication support other than Detrol or self help rescues. Have you checked with your MD about medication for pain for this rough time? Most prescription pain medications cannot be used when you are driving or working. As strong as we recommend in the clinic, a prescribed medication, Ultracet (2) also sold as Tramadol that would take the edge off your pain so you can sleep and your body as well as your bladder would get the message to relax so sleep would be undisturbed.

This brings me to the question - is Detrol LA helping or are you having difficulty starting to void? Experience has taught us that anti-cholinergic such as Detrol often can cause problems at a flare time by setting up retention reaction meaning you having difficulty or cannot start to void.

I have written about these rescues before but have you tried lidocaine cream (without a prescription) or the prescription form of lidocaine that is an ointment and lasts longer when applied to the perineum and then wrapped ice packs. This gives a sense of relief so that you can again rest.

You also mentioned you purchased Prelief to take before meals. The company states it should used be three times a day before meals as a mild anti-acid working on reducing acid in foods.

Also there is a nonprescription analgesic and antiseptic for urine called AZO. The prescription form is Pyridium (phenozopridine) also known as urogesic or Urelle. All three produce urine that is either orange or blue green. And can be used for 2 to 3 days as a rescue. Suggested use during a flare time and especial before bedtime.

And most specifically to make sure you do not have urinary (UTI) infection. Chances are you do not, but a sample of your urine should be sent to the lab for culture.

JO

From: Jan
To: support@icaction.com
Sent: Thursday, Mar 6, at 3:45 PM
Re: Physicians, etc.

Help, I am miserable. Being intimate is difficult.

Jan

From: support@icaction.com
To: Jan
Sent: Thursday, Mar 6, at 5:45 PM
Re: Physicians, etc.

Jan:

If you were a coach and a player were injured you would advise:

1. First ice packs
2. Fluids
3. Activity – stretching not pounding
4. The best support shoes for work and play
5. Lying down when you can
6. Sexual intercourse - often pelvic pain comes afterward and just as a bruise persists after an injury. Voiding pre and post intercourse.
7. Rinse perineal area with baking soda and cool water
8. LUBRICATION – Astroglide has had good reports because of its smoothness that lasts. Local gynecologist suggested Extra Virgin Olive Oil (EVOO) A use that Rachel Ray does not have in her recipe books – yet. There are some who have reported using vitamin E oil. Problem seems to be that it is bit sticky.
9. Room temperature is not body. All lubricants need to be warmed slightly.
10. Back to #1 – Ice pack after intercourse.

From your emails, you are hitting a lot of the marks that push a flare.

When is your spring break?

JO

From: support@icaction.com
To: Jan
Sent: On Friday, Mar 7, at 8:59 AM
Re: Physicians, etc.

Jan:

1. The more you worry, the more adrenalin you pump and the more adrenalin you pump the sensation for pain is heightened for most of us.

2. That is why often an anxiety medication is prescribed like Ativan (Valium), Xanax, Lorezapan are used on as needed bases and an antidepressant that deals with serotonin loss as Zoloft are part of the medication initial mix.

3. Sounds like I work in a pharmacy, but IC is a condition that initially is often in a run away state and more often then not each symptom needs to be evaluated for how much it plays into the misery increase – Stress – is a big player – If only we sat on the porch and had punch delivered to us on a silver tray as we watched the sail boats go by. Now that personally would drive me crazy in ten minutes, but my body often needs just that. – To slow down.

Activities

4. What has helped is running activities in a Lycra material shorts or light-weight girdle that supports you mid section and pelvic area. Not too tight but gives a sense of holding the pelvic region up and in. Not the entire solution but you might consider what clothing you wear when you are in your physical activities. This includes the hours you spend on your feet and lifting in the classroom.

5. Also the problem with soccer and street running is uneven surfaces and the variation of give to the surface. Again the pounding. Best running shoes you can buy for hard terrain – changed every 3 months if you wear them regularly even if they look like they are perfect. Core protection is what you want.

6. Post activity, ice down. Advil (anti-inflammatory properties) and if the wind is blowing and the grass is growing, an antihistamine before the activity can help.

7. Most of us learn our limits and then we can weigh the pros and cons of pushing them. First order of business is to get out of the IC flare that is winning your personal 10K.

I will be out of town until 21 March. Will check emails, but not sure how often I will get a chance to respond. Please keep the emails coming if this of value to you.

JO

From: Jan
To: support@icaction.com
Sent: On Friday, Mar 7, at 4:42 PM
Re: Protection from Trauma

Jo:

Thank you for your response about sports. You gave me hope and some useful information that I don't have to give up everything I love because of this injury to my bladder.

I am planning on laying off soccer for a week and just walking instead to see if it improves the situation. I would like to see more improvement than I have been with my organic diet. The soccer I play is on a rubberized AstroTurf and any running I do is on a treadmill. Even though it isn't hard concrete, it seems that it could be delaying the healing at this point.

I am grateful for all your experience and communication with me. It is all so new to me, and hopefully what I learn will help me speed up the healing process.

Jan

From: support@icaction.com
To: Jan
Sent: Friday, Mar 7, at 7:30 PM
Re: I have made almost every mistake in the book

Jan:

First thing I learned is that it took time for me to reach my negative physical state and it was going to take time to undo the destruction. That was a hard lesson.

Did you know that IC has other names? Like "Teachers' Bladders and Nurses Bladders" Mmmm wonder why?

I remember an email of a teacher who said one of the pleasures she had to give up was coffee with the other teachers early in the AM or she would spend the entire day with the heightened urge and frequency. She found she could sip on herbal tea and be a part of the group she so enjoyed. So it was not giving some thing up – it was a matter of adapting.

Please do stretching exercises and start before you get out of bed in the AM and before bedtime. We could learn from cats – stretch.

The up side of all of this is that you begin to learn to treat your body with more respect and you pass the message on to your family. Don't I sound wise?

JO

From: Jan
To: support@icaction.com
Sent: Sunday, Mar 9, at 7:49 AM
Re: I have made almost every mistake in the book

Jo:

Thank you for your note, I had not heard of the other names. I can see that this will take time to figure out.

I took an hour car ride to hike a nature reserve with a girl friend yesterday. It was such a great place in terms of people and the beautiful scenery. I came home singing and feeling much more relaxed. But after the car trip my left buttock was pretty painful even though I sat on an extra pillow. My thoughts had been to put an ice pack on during the drive back, but I was kind of embarrassed about it when riding with my friend.

Today I am paying for it. Woke up early and my pelvis was aching. Had to cancel a trip to my kids' track meet that would have been an hour and a half car trip one way. My husband was able to take them, but I hate not being there to see them.

I am wondering what the procedures are for traveling. I went online and read about heating pads, sitting at a pelvic tilt on a padded cushion, and you suggested Advil after working out.

Do you have any travel suggestions? My kids have several more away track meets, and my family is planning to go skiing during the spring vacation coming up at the end of March. I am not looking forward to the 4-hour car trip to the mountains.

I guess yesterday I could have used ice on the way down and on the way up and taken an Advil? I felt great during the moderate hike up and down the hillsides. It was the car ride that seemed to cause the discomfort.

I am confused about heat versus ice pack. Is it an individual thing, or is there a medical recommendation?

Since you are away, I am hoping you are taking a great trip somewhere traveling in comfort.

Jan

From: support@icaction.com
To: Jan
Sent: Sunday, Mar 9, at 11:29 AM
Re: Travel Suggestions

Question - Any chance there is a gluteus muscle pull or nerve irritation from walking an irregular terrain and a re injury of the same area? How much stretching did you do before you took off for your walk? A car trip alone can tighten up the muscles everywhere – arms included. Any chance this is not one that is directly bladder connected?

Each time we say 'ouch' is an opportunity to learn what we can do and when we have pushed too far. The activities that can be chosen have to have some planning.

Travel

The bladder is multi layered muscular organ or it couldn't squeeze as effectively as it does. So pulling out the iced gel pack for local relief and to minimize damage is a good idea no matter what the cause. Saying that the bladder becomes inflamed muscle groups because of IC is very true.

Simple rule – inflammation is injury, inflammation has a release of mast cells causing swelling, whether it is from a sunburn, bug bite, muscle pull. Internal or external, ice reduces swelling and by extension reduces pain that would be caused by the swelling.

When you travel by car a small cooler with gel ice packs, is part of your travel kit.

Drinking water when you travel makes you stop to void and also to stretch every two hours or so is good for everyone. A contoured seat cushion - usually foam or gel - is great to support your back and buttocks and that means your pelvic organs.

The worst are airplane seats. I ask for two small airplane pillows - one for the small of my back and one to sit one. These days you bring your own or it costs about 8 dollars for small pillow and blanket pack. Have seen blow up rings that are of some value.

I use to take my ice gel packs with me, but these days with the bag checks it has become a hassle so I take sandwich size zip locks and ask the attendant for ice and double bag it and put on my lap. I have even used a cold bottle of water for pelvic relief when traveling. I wrap it in a hand towel I take with me. I have learned that for me any trip over 90 minutes means ice. From my experience, there is more than a few times that once I settle into the travel rhythm the urgency and frequency subside. This leads me to believe that stress is pushing more than a few nerve buttons.

If you have low back pain - and that is most of us with IC - if your car or SUV has a built in seat warmer it is the best for traveling to use when traveling to have on as insurance or to help low back pain. Again this is a muscle spasm tension because of bladder spasms.

Inflammation – cool it down. Spasms – warm it up.

JO

From: Jan
To: support@icaction.com
Sent: Sunday, Mar 16, at 9:30 AM
Re: Local Doctor

Jo:

How are you?

I was relieved to find a doctor in this area who has experience working with IC patients and is aware of Elmiron treatment. His name is Dr. C. They also have clinics in the 4 surrounding areas.

Dr. C. said there are about 75 to 100 patients with IC in this area he has dealt with, and a nurse tried to start a support group, and it didn't work out.

After hearing about my symptoms and giving me a physical exam of my urethra, vaginal area, he has me on the following program for 6 weeks until the next visit:

1. Detrol LA for the bladder spasms – 1 pill daily
2. Prescription antihistamine – Hydroxyzine HCL 10 mg tablet before bedtime. I noticed from the medical handouts that this also treats anxiety.
3. Prescription for physical therapy to treat the pelvic aching (pelvic dysfunction) – a couple of women therapist have had a lot of success with this therapy treatment of pelvic massage. I should have my first appointment in the next week or two.
4. Limit exercise to stretching, weight lifting, and try the elliptical (until next visit) - no jumping or running.
5. Continue watching foods to find out what triggers me - he didn't stress organic – but still think it is an important thing not to put any more toxins through the bladder than necessary. I do have a biochemist friend who tests produce for many large growers in the local area. She is dubious about much difference in organic, and non-organic produce. She said she rarely finds more than 5% pesticide reside on regular produce, and organic farmers can use up to 5%. Interesting....
6. Deal with stress – I am lying down more! And I took the morning off from work to meet with this doctor as soon as possible to get some help.

He wants me to wait until my next visit to see how I am doing before he prescribes the Elmiron. I am a little nervous about that because I want to heal besides deal with the symptoms. I am much relieved to have found a local doctor to help and have been in a much better mood.

Hope you are doing well.

Jan

From: Jan
To: support@icaction.com
Sent: Tuesday, Mar 18, at 6:23 PM
Re: Local Doctor

Jo:

Did you get the email about the doctor I found?

I just met with the physical therapist for pelvic dysfunction, and she was encouraging. She has been working with IC patients for four years in this area with success in helping alleviate the symptoms.

My task at this point is to use a biofeedback device to do Kegel type contractions and releases. It is supposed to retrain that area to function properly so I don't develop incontinence. I have other exercises to strengthen the abdominal wall and some stretches. I'm not sure what else she will be doing and this was basically the first visit with an examination and paperwork to fill out.

She is very interested in your clinic so I will give her your address.

Hope all is well.

Jan

From: support@icaction.com
To: Jan
Sent: Saturday, Mar 22, at 5:24 PM
Re: Local Doctor

Jan:

Will be interested in your progress with the PT.

The reports we have had with pelvic floor dysfunction PT is relaxation with vaginal massage and the pelvic floor spasms are released = less pain.

Kegels have been reported to cause distress (pain) if you are having a flare of any degree.

We have not had any success in having pelvic floor physical therapy covered by insurance and so the equipment and services are very limited in our area. Please remember that the spasms are a symptom of inflammation so your medication diet, rest, etc. continue the healing and pain control.

It is a trust issue for most women when they take this PT path - a matter of speaking up if and when you are uncomfortable.

JO

From: support@icaction.com
To: Jan
Sent: Saturday, Mar 22, at 7:00 PM
Re: Local Doctor

Jan:

Reviewing my emails from the beginning.

Glad you found a local resource for medical support.

Elmiron takes 3 to 6 months orally to cover the damage that has been done over the months and years to your bladder lining.

The hydroxyzine – Atarax is an old time antihistamine (works and is economical). It can make you sleepy when you first take it. We say take it about two hours before bedtime so you do not have a hangover in the morning.

Over time you may need higher doses depending on your weight and sensitivity to the medication.

You did not mention and often prescribed medication. Elavil/amitriptyline usually 10 mg to start is for bladder spasms and in much higher dose of 100 mg it can be used for anxiety control. Have not heard of Atarax used for anxiety control recently, but it use to be used as a preoperative sedation; like Benadryl it is an antihistamine that has as an effect causing sleepiness.

A note to remember – if you feel the hydroxyzine/Atarax is causing you to feel tired ask the MD to switch to an antihistamine like Allegra or Claritin that does not give the sleepy feeling.

Please know that over the counter varieties of most medications as a general rule has less potency than the prescription form.

Also, before I left, you asked about a tush cushion – I get catalogs with recommendations for bottom and back support cushions. Wonder if a Bed Bath and Beyond-type store might sell them? Purchased my auto seat cushion from Wal-Mart automotive section.

JO

From: Jan
To: support@icaction.com
Sent: Sunday, Mar 23, at 6:05 AM
Re: Local Doctor

Jo:

I am happy to hear you were able to travel to Florida and back.

Thank you for your response. As always, I really value your experience and suggestions.

I am having a hard time reducing this flare. I have been eating organically and avoiding acid triggers. I didn't think Prelief was doing much, but when I ran out, I had more burning sensation in my urethra… so now I know it does help me.

I am having aching a lot of the time, especially by mid afternoon or even mornings when I wake up. I have been using Tylenol and icing after walking. The walking is even making me ache more.

I am stopping Kegel exercises since I notice more aching since I started. I hope I can get some of the massage, and I will need to see if my health insurance will cover it.

I was worried that the Dr. wanted me to wait a month for Elmiron. I am not sure why, except he wanted to see how I was doing on the antihistamine.

Would you recommend a stronger dose of antihistamine or a different one? I think I need something right now to help with anxiety.

I decided to stay home to rest and try to get another appointment to change the meds or up the strength while my family goes on a 4-day skiing trip. I really wanted to go with them, but the 4-hour car trip and lack of fridge in the hotel room for my food didn't seem workable at this point.

Please advise me on what to do. I am concerned that I am not feeling some relief from the aching.

Jan

From: support@icaction.com
To: Jan
Sent: Sunday, Mar 23, at 11:11 AM
Re: Anxiety and Small Victories

Jan:

Pain produces anxiety because we feel out of control, and we physically are. Add pelvic pain to the demands of the rest of our lives, and it feels like we are riding a run away horse.

Since you are so articulate about your stress symptoms – would suggest a call to your primacy MD or Urologist and ask about antidepressants such as Zoloft or one of the many other serotonin uptake inhibitors.

Reasons: We need serotonin. Pain and stress can drain it away faster than we can replace it when we are dealing with stress or any kind.

These specific antidepressants medications slow down that process so our bodies can catch-up.

Zoloft, as an example, has a starter pack of 25 mg for 7 days, and then it goes up to 50 mg. It takes about 7 to 10 days to stabilize the amount in your blood stream. One pill per day. I have worked with women who were so frazzled they could not add up 2+2.

You are dealing with nerve pain sending a cascade of pain messages to your brain, and it is on overload. As you have learned quickly, you know your body best and are your best advocate.

Yes, you can increase the antihistamine with your doctor's blessing, but your MD probably thinks that the antihistamine will calm down the mast cells/histamine release and by extension reduce inflammation and then the pain.

But because of the multiple facets to nerve fibers, this is only one part of the recovery process. Our office usually has oral prescriptions for IC or: Elmiron (pentosan poly sulfate sodium), Elavil (amitriptyline), Atarax (hydroxyzine), and often a course of Zoloft (sertraline Hcl) until the pain subsides. Then reevaluate about the use of a medication like Detrol LA if needed or if it does not add to symptom problems with inability to start to void. There are multiple variations on these medications dosages and brands, etc. but this is the beginning suggestion list to discuss with your urologist.

Go to ICaction.com and on one link is to a diet log to print. This has been the best initial tool to track pain symptoms over 24 hours.

Would encourage you to do so for 3 days and see what your diet, pain, fluid intake, voiding/BM pattern is.

Pain scale is 1 to 10 – 1to 3 tolerable – 4 and 5 hard to tolerate (self rescues as baking soda, AZO) - *I bet you still go to work.* 6+ not going to work and an ER visit for pain relief.

Right now suspend reality for a short while with a cup of vanilla tea and a Russell Crow movie, like "A Good Year."

Jo

From: Jan
To: support@icaction.com
Sent: Sunday, Mar 23, at 12:10:11 PM
Re: Anxiety and Small Victories

Jo:

Thank you for your fast reply. I remember in your first email telling me that you were limiting info since it was more than one can absorb at one time.

I am glad you keep repeating and clarifying basics right now. You are really my guide at this point, with my body giving me the feedback.

I will follow up on your suggestions.

Thank you so much for all you support.

From: Jan
To: support@icaction.com
Sent: Tuesday, Mar 25, at 8:06 AM
Re: Flare – resolving?

Jo:

I have spent the last 3 days pretty much sitting, and the pelvic aching is much better. I need to slowly start adding more movement back in, I guess. The first day when I tried to take a walk, it flared back up. I guess the trick now is to start slowly and back into more movement?

I have an appointment to talk to my primary care MD about antidepressant you mentioned this week, and rescheduled with my urologist to request Elmiron. He is out on vacation until the first week of April.

Do you still have flares, or is that pretty much under control with your treatment and meds and diet?

Jan

From: support@icaction.comJan
To: Jan
Sent: Tuesday, Mar 25, at 1:35 PM
Re: Question is how much can you test the limits?

Jan:

Happy that your body is settling down after a rough time.

Motherly advice:

It is human nature to do too much when there is a break in the pain cycle, i.e. the gentleman I interviewed who was doing well and decided to move a piano – not a good idea – or the woman who went out and cut 2 acres of grass (she didn't think it would matter since she was on a riding mower.)

A easy neighborhood walk is preferable to a run.

Yes, I can wake the sleeping dragon of IC, mainly stressing out or neglecting to eat with long periods of no food between. But I now know the signs of body neglect and change my ways more quickly than I use to. Also I do not want to neglect to say I had a bladder lift surgery (big babies, gravity, weight gain, and time.) This was a great help in not having urine remaining in my bladder. I was beyond Kegel help and in my opinion most of us are.

My I suggest a pressure-free gel cushion for work or in your auto. You can find many different types found online.

JO

From: Jan
To: support@icaction.com
Sent: Wednesday, Mar 26, at 1:54 PM
Re: Moving Forward

Jo:

Yesterday, instead of my 25 min. hike around the neighborhood up and down hills, I took a 15 min. walk a few blocks away and back. Did OK and made sure I iced afterwards.

Today took a shopping trip and walked about an hour. Wow, at that point my hip area was very tired, but improved when I stopped and stood still, and after I came home, sat down and iced. It's progress, and

I can see how tempting it would be to go back and try full blast. I'm just happy not to have constant aching. So my goal right now is to keep trying little bits and resting a lot!

This spring break has been very helpful. I am wondering how it will go when I am back in the classroom next week and trying to take care of the family needs too?

I do have an appointment April 8 to request Elmiron. I hope between summer and the Elmiron, I can be in a better place by next fall.

Jan

From: support@icaction.com
To: Jan
Sent: Thursday, Mar 27, at 3:02 PM
Re: Thank you for checking in

Jan:

I bet the most difficult part for you is doing less – doing more is a snap compared to take a breath.

Think I spoke about stretching. The best - Yoga as a learned discipline that also is a great help to reduce stress. If you have a parks and recreation department, YWCA, or community college continuing education they is usually a beginning class.

Are you up for a massage? You discussed the pelvic floor treatments, but a day spa with a massage therapist is worth a try.

JO

From: Jan
To: support@icaction.com
Sent: Thursday, Mar 27, at 6:25 PM
Re: Thank you for checking in

Jo:

Thanks for the reminder of what I can do right now. I am fighting the urge to do more....I really feel like I am turning into a marshmallow.

There is a Tai Chi class and some yoga in this area though the local programs. I can see doing that, but am concerned about keeping the aerobic aspect up some how for heart health. Any suggestions?

What are you able to do for yourself?

Jan

From: support@icaction.com
To: Jan
Sent: Thursday, Mar 27, at 10:00 PM
Re: It is all about the elliptical

Jan:

Simple answer is working out on a recumbent bike or elliptical trainer.

JO

APRIL

From: support@icaction.com
To: Jan
Sent: Saturday, Apr 26, at 5:05 PM
Re: It is all about the elliptical

Always hope that no news is good news. How are you doing? JO

From: Jan
To: support@icaction.com
Sent: Sunday, Apr 27, at 6:30:06 PM
Re: Jan – Checking in

Hi, Jo:

Thank you for your note.

I started Elmiron about 2 ½ weeks ago, and I am sticking to the organic diet, Prelief the antihistamine and 100 mg of Zoloft per day. So I hope this is the best treatment for the symptoms and healing.

It is difficult for me not to move on a daily basis. I can see what you were saying about over doing it when you start to feel better.

I don't have the aching all day anymore, but I try to take a walk daily up and down the hills of the neighborhood, I start feeling achy afterwards. I am using ice afterwards. I am so restless and frustrated, but grateful I am doing better than I was.

So now it is time to wait for the Elmiron to help with the healing process.

The physical therapy sometimes relaxes me and sometimes doesn't. If we use a heating pad for 10 min., and than the therapist massages my groin muscles that seems to be the most relaxing.

My lifestyle is so sedentary to what I was used to. I hope it is temporary.

I hope all is well.

Jan

JUNE

From: Jan
To: support@icaction.com
Sent: Sunday, Jun 1, at 4:18 PM
Re: Lyme disease

Hi, Jo:

I am wondering if anyone at your clinic or in your experience has had a connection made between IC symptoms and Lyme disease.

I got a tick bite, which developed the big circular rash about a year before my Bartholin cyst and all the following symptoms. The local doctor treated me for about 3 weeks with an antibiotic. But I was wondering if that is what could have started all this? Jan

From: support@icaction.com
To: Jan
Sent: Thursday, Jun 5, at 8:23 PM
Re: Lyme disease

Spoke to Ed (Dr. Davis) and he said there is no published link. But Lyme is like all diseases, activates the immune system, and we really do not know what it leaves behind.

There are reports of IC in males and females after courses of the acne treatment drug, Accutane. It changes the body's chemical balance and produces a drying affect.

I have heard patients in the practice who swear that after a hysterectomy their IC symptoms occurred. Now was that because there was latex catheter use, antibiotics, or discovery that the pelvic pain was caused by the bladder and not or not only by the reproductive organs? Know that IC is often found in post radiation and chemotherapy patients after treatment for cancer.

So is IC a body reaction to an invasion of disease or treatment or a genetic predisposition to that brings about the bladder cells struggle to be repaired and replaced?

Fibro, Irritable Bowel Syndrome (IBS), Migraines, and IC all seem to have links and all are an inflammatory process. I realize every day how little we really know about the entire process. So we deal with the symptoms. How are you doing? Jo

From: Jan
To: support@icaction.com
Sent: Tuesday, Jun 10, at 7:18 AM
Re: Research

Hi, Jo:

Thank you for your research about my question of Lyme disease possibly causing IC.

I am doing okay. I just finished my last week of school with a lot of extra pressure. I did a good job the weekend I was home doing report cards, in balancing housework, rest, and all the paper work. It went very well.

I am able to take a walk daily, on the hilly route, which before bothered me. I did have more pelvic discomfort when I took a walk up a steep hill while I was out camping with my son and the cub scouts for one night. The car trip was 45 minutes and okay.

So I can see progress. It seems very slow, but I am grateful for it.

I have a friend who just completed a 6 day Pelvic Pain Clinic in Santa Rosa California. It is based on 8 years of research by Stanford University and teaches relaxation methods and trigger points to massage by yourself or your partner. There is a book out that I have ordered. It is titled "Headache in the Pelvis" by Dr. Wise and Dr. Anderson.

I am continuing the physical therapy with Sam. It seems to help in keeping the muscles relaxed. I have also been trying some yoga classes and find that most of it is okay except deep lunges on the left side that seems to increase discomfort on that side.

Always looking for more information to help!

Thank you again for your continuing conversations with me.

Jan

From: support@icaction.com
To: Jan
Sent: Wednesday, Jun 25, at 8:04 PM
Re: IC, pharmaceutical clinical trials, the future

Jan:

Thank you for the information about the pain clinic. How are you doing?

I was out of town and had 200 emails, and your latest one was missed. Please excuse me. I sadly have learned that giving my email address when ordering from a catalog is now added to my list of lifetime mistakes.

IC and pelvic pain

Recently IC had the addition of more initials to better describe the symptom pattern, Bladder Pain Syndrome (BPS). This is an acknowledgement that there is more to bladder-generated pain than one organ.

The pharmaceutical company, Pfizer, has FDA approval and markets oral medication, Lyrica for Fibromyalgia (muscle/nerve) pain. Lyrica has been used off label (meaning with patients knowledge they be prescribed a medication that is not been approved by the FDA for a specific disease but appears to work for the control of symptoms. We have had success with Lyrica for pelvic pain of bladder original for several years. Hopefully a company like Pfizer will have a clinical trial for a formulation like Lyrica like to control IC pelvic pain.

Lilly and Pfizer are also looking into infusions (Intravenous) routes of medication delivery that are based on controlling the growth of pain fibers. The research part of the urology office is involved in both clinical trials.

This research into nerve fibers recruitment is very important because the problem has been that Elmiron may cover the thinned or missing bladder protective lining, but then the pain fibers (C fibers) are already activated and after an unknown length of activation time do not know how to turn themselves off even when the bladder lining appears to be healed.

It is indeed a syndrome. More than one moving part.

It would be great for BPS/IC to finally have a pharmaceutical advocate that recognizes a medical problem. I am banking on the pharmaceutical philosophy of "find a medication that meets a symptom need, and they will come." Meaning the medical profession will recognize a real disease process. With or without a laboratory test, BPS/IC will be recognized and there will be logical and systemic treatment. The hit and often miss treatment of IC is not good medicine.

JO

From: Jan
To: support@icaction.com
Sent: Wednesday, Jun 25, at 8:04 PM
Re: Catching up

Hi, Jo:

Glad to hear you are finding more possible medical support for IC people.

I am doing better on and off. A week ago, quite a bit of pelvic aching which probably went along with walking every day. Got a bladder infection and besides the antibiotic, got some Pyridium (painkiller) which seemed to relieve the pelvic aching some what even with a 4-hour car trip for my daughter's club soccer tournament.

I am experimenting with a yoga routine as soon as I wake up. Seems to help with the minor pelvic ache I wake up with. I will see what happens when I add walking back in a week.

What a great day! I was finally able to eat some mayonnaise without any burning. I did take Prelief first as usual. Almost two months on the Elmiron

Thanks for your email.

Jan

From: support@icaction.com
To: Jan
Sent: Thursday, Jun 26, at 9:15 AM
Re: Only one question

Jan:

The bladder infection diagnosis – was a urine request for a culture sent to the lab for confirmation?

Or was your urine production cloudy with a strong scent along with the increased urge, frequency and perhaps burning. Jo

From: Jan
To: support@icaction.com
Sent: Thursday, Jun 26, at 11:54 AM
Re: Reply

Jo:

My urine sample was looked at and determined to be full of bacteria according to the primary care office I was at. The only symptom I noticed was some slight discomfort when I urinated which was not usual for me. I think I might have set myself up for it by trying to apply some Vaseline in that area before I went into a chlorinated pool last week. (Something I read about on the IC site)

Since the antibiotics, feeling better

Why did you ask?

Jan

From: support@icaction.com
To: Jan
Sent: Thursday, Jun 26, at 1:52 PM
Re: Urine tests and infections

Jan:

Short answer "Too many antibiotics"

Antibiotics set the stage for vaginal yeast infections, diarrhea, and development of drug resistant super germs. If you are not lactose sensitive, think real yogurt, sour cream, or use acidophilus tablets, like the brand Lactinex, when taking antibiotics. Plus there is diminishing the list of antibiotics that will work to control infection when and if you do become ill because of bacteria. This has become a huge problem in the US.

When the physician sends a specimen to the lab for *culture and sensitivity* (C&S) the lab can tell if it is contaminant or if there is an organism requiring treatment - what is and what antibiotic is appropriate for treating the bacteria starting from the <u>least</u> powerful antibiotic.

Clean catch urine specimens are notorious for being wrong. In the office, we all do a simple strip test or use a test process that reports a series of informative results, i.e. is there glucose or sugar, blood, nitrites, etc. in your urine. If there is blood or red cells (often invisible to the eye) white cells, nitrites it signals the physician to send the specimen to the lab for more accurate testing – the *culture* part. When the lab determines what antibiotic needs to be prescribed that is the *sensitivity* part.

As a female, you get more urine on your hand than you do in the collection cup. With IC, you can have white cells and red blood cell, even if you cannot see any trace of either and your urine looks clear. And to this day most physicians and emergency rooms, including urologist, think <u>infection</u> and <u>not IC</u> when a red blood cell shows up. Reporting an increase of urgency and frequency also points to an infection, but with IC you have to also think this may be a flare not in need of an antibiotic.

Nitrites showing up as active on a test strip are better sign of infection. These are the source of the intense smell and cloudy urine that are often accompanying the urge and frequency increase.

Short version – have the physician's office send your specimen to the lab for a double check, before you take antibiotics. This procedure takes about 2 days to find out if there are bacteria and another day (3 total) for the lab to report back if there are bacteria that need antibiotic treatment and which antibiotics is the organism sensitive to.

With IC – white cells and red blood cells are always being sloughed off the injured bladder lining and an increase in urge, frequency, and pelvic pain mixed in signals a flare of some degree and the antibiotics have little to do with you feeling better – It is a medication placebo affect. If told we have a bladder infection or urinary track infection (UTI), we all begin to drink more water and rest a bit more so a flare has a chance of subsiding and too often antibiotics are given credit for a job they never need to be called upon to do.

The prescription brand called Pyridium or Urelle are two examples that act as antispasmodics and analgesics that soothes the bladder lining and urethral area when you void; an over the counter example is the brand AZO.

As a bedtime rescue, while waiting for lab results, we advise keeping it on hand or if you know a flare might be lurking take a Pyridium tablet before bedtime so your sleep and may not be troubled with the multiple needs to void because of feeling irritated during the night.

If you noticed you need to flush the toilet quickly. Its bright orange tie dye hue stains and you might need a pant liner that you change frequently for hygiene and to lower the risk of causing a bladder infection because of contamination of E. coli.

JO

From: support@icaction.com
To: Jan
Sent: Thursday, Jun 26, at 1:54 PM
Re: Pools and Spas

Jan:

Pools and spas - Best to rinse off as soon as you get out of the pool or spa. The chlorine is bathing your entire body and with a spa you are warm and the pores and blood vessels are dilated especially of your urethra, vagina, and perineal area is exposed to chemicals. If you have some baking soda put it on a washcloth with the water and use as a wipe down to neutralize the chlorine.

JO

From: Jan
To: support@icaction.com
Sent: Friday, Jun 27, at 1:36 PM
Re: Latest info

Thank you for the information. I did tell the doctor about the IC condition. Shows how much education needs to be done in the field with patients and the medical profession.

I liked the tip also for pools and spas.

Do you have any tips about what to try eating or drinking when you are getting over the stomach bug? I used to try the ginger ale and saltine regimen, but don't think that would be so good with the diet restrictions... Have been sick the last couple of days.

Jan

From: support@icaction.com
To: Jan
Sent: Saturday, Jun 28, at 9:00 PM
Re: Help with what to drink if have the flu

Jan:

Hope you are improving.

The ICA recommends the brand sparkling water Perrier and it seems to be okay. Saltine crackers have baking soda in them. I do not have a problem with Canada Dry ginger ale, but Vernors brand is a bit much for me. Also fall back to my vanilla tea. I am big on pear juice frozen in cubes and used to make the water or Perrier has a bit of favor. Also the choice of no monosodium glutamate (MSG), organic chicken broths have appeared in the soup aisles. MSG plays havoc with an IC bladder.

JO

From: Jan
To: support@icaction.com
Sent: Monday, Jun 30, at 7:57 AM
Re: Improved from upset stomach

Jo:

Finally feeling better and starting to eat more food.

I found that plain baked potatoes and apples with the skin were doable.

I can't wait to get some Perrier and pear juice. I am so bored with drinking water and milk all the time. Have started drinking some peppermint and chamomile tea. By the way what vanilla tea is okay?

Jan

From: support@icaction.com
To: Jan
Sent: Monday, Jun 30, at 7:57 AM
Re: Vanilla tea

Glad you are improving.

Have had great success with vanilla tea – was recommended by a patient about 2 years ago. And the big point is that it tastes like drinking something instead of water.

Have not had it iced but bet it would be good.

JO

JULY

From: Jan
To: support@icaction.com
Sent: Sunday, Jul 13, at 8:31 PM
Re: Vanilla tea

The good news is that my last urine sample was clean and no trace of blood. The bad news is that I did get a yeast infection and even secondary bacteria because the good bacteria got killed off from the antibiotics for the bladder infection. So now the next round of medication to treat that, and I am taking probiotic acidophilus on my own and trying to limit the sugars.

I am finding that I am also able to eat more foods than earlier with a reaction ... making progress.

A woman underwent the "Stanford Protocol" program going to my physical therapist. I will be interested to see how she trains Sammy (physical therapist) to work with the muscle trigger points that is part of their treatment. I had Sammy do an internal massage for the first time, and she did find lots of tight muscles areas. It was not real comfortable but it showed me the need for it.

Hope you are having some time off this summer to enjoy the beautiful weather.

Jan

From: support@icaction.com
To: Jan
Sent: Wednesday, Jul 16, at 8:05 AM
Re: Yeast infection and history

Jan:

Back home after a short trip to Catalina.

Glad to hear that your bladder is back to cooperating with the rest of your busy life. I assume you have been on Monistat or Diflucan for the yeast infection.

Both have miconazole nitrate as the active ingredient to cure vaginal yeast infections.

If you are not lactose intolerant, now would be a great time to hit the "real" yogurt and sour cream products. Monistat rids you of the yeast, but you need to replenish the good bacteria. In addition, a good bacteria food regimen for at least one bottles worth of a product like Lactinex (acidophilus) or Align that is sold over the counter but stored in the refrigerator of the pharmacy because it has more active ingredients than the usual shelf stored products. Another watchword is probiotic.

Just like the antibiotic went through your entire body it deleted the needed bacteria in your entire system, gastrointestinal included.

Question – For my own thought processes about IC – can you please tell me about your UTI experience?

The original ID bladder infection – was your urine cloudy and with a strong odor and/or did you have an increase in urinary misery symptoms, urge, frequency, burning, visual blood, and the organism isolated – E coli or?

Thank you, JO

From: **Jan**
To: support@icaction.com
Sent: **Wednesday, Jul 23, at 9:16 AM**
Re: **Yeast infection report**

Jo:

Just got back from a camping trip with my son and than had a 3-day upset stomach…glad that's over.

Thank you for the info about acidophilus products. I am half way through a bottle of probiotic to rebuild the healthy bacteria.

I really don't have too much information for you about the UTI experience. There were a couple of things that could have triggered the UTI… if that's what it was.

I did apply Vaseline at the spa but forgot and went back to front. Also had painful intercourse that week with a lot of discomfort on the left side. The symptom that made me seek treatment was a slight feeling of pain when I started urinating. I didn't seem to have an odor until I did get a mild yeast infection after the darned antibiotics. I should have started the acidophilus at the same time as the antibiotic.

The doctor gave me one pill to take care of the yeast (Diflucan). I am going back to the gynecologist office today to have them check which kind of yeast… I usually have a more difficult strain to get rid of.

Hope this info gives you some ideas.

Catalina…hope you had a great time

Jan

From: support@icaction.com
To: Jan
Sent: Friday, Jul, 25 at 11:21 AM
Re: **Could it have been a flare?**

Warning: Turned into a long email and there maybe some pearls of wisdom repeated

Jan:

It is definitely a busy summer and it sounds like you have not missed a beat with activities.

My question is how has your family activity list affected your BPS (Bladder Pain Syndrome) or as it is now showing up in the literature BPS/IC?

Question: Was it an IC flare rather than a UTI?

As an example on your activity list included sexual intercourse. A big symptom is one to set up the urethritis sensation or pelvic pain more often reported to the right but can be to left side of your lower abdomen above your bikini line. And that also means possibly having pain circle under toward the back under your rib cage. Throw in low back pain on the misery PBS stack. This is why sexual intimacy is often an overwhelming issue.

Flare producer – sexual intercourse: Think running a 10K in high heels.

Now this email gets long.

Urethral discomfort usually is connected directly to inflammation - either caused internally by IC and/or bacteria but often by friction of intercourse, clothing, sitting, standing, running.

Time to think loose clothing and better yet no underpants and a loose dress or skirt when you are at home. Baking soda rinse before and after intercourse or a day of running around needs iced gel pack to the perineum at sleep time, or when you get a chance to rest and watching TV or reading, etc.

One suggestion from a gynecologist; if that is a sensitive and is overwhelmed, use a hair dryer on NO heat to dry after a shower or voiding to keep contact with tissue or towels or clothing at a minimum. All this helps resolve the urethral discomfort whether the inflammation is caused by IC, friction, bacteria, yeast, or chemical exposure

Also there is over the counter lidocaine cream – one brand is LMX 4% - cost around $25.00. There is a 5% prescription product that has an ointment base so it lasts longer, but the OTC cream is very helpful for the urethral discomfort post intercourse or any strenuous physical activity. Then you can add the rescue measures listed to help resolve the uncomfortable or worse urethral discomfort/pain.

Lubrication is so necessary for sexual intercourse. Even with lust, lubrication is a must. Astroglide with the least amount of additives, we found, to be the best for helping prepare the vagina. It is a matter of not hurting so that sexual pleasure can at least be a feeling of closeness. One local gynecologist offered extra virgin olive oil as his non-allergic choice for vaginal lubrication.

Also a good suggestion is a prescription medication to have on hand like Urelle, or Pyridium for before or directly after intercourse as part of a flare rescue kit. Urelle is like Pyridium and AZO (OTC), but your urine turns pale blue-green instead of orange. We have recommended it as a possibility to be used as a pre- or post-intercourse medication because of the soothing properties as when it is used because of a UTI.

Possible UTI?

I have not had a chance to review our all your past emails so excuse me if I have written this before.

A confusing issue with BPS/IC is our thought process breaking away from the remedy of using antibiotics for every increase in urinary symptoms, burning, increased urge, increased frequency, and post intercourse urethral discomfort. So many physicians continue to follow the tradition that if an office lab test shows any white cells, red cells or nitrites the conclusion is reached that it must be a Urinary Tract Infection (UTI) therefore an antibiotic needs to be the prescription of medical intervention. No need for a laboratory analysis is the rule under this standard of care.

To prove the point, our office sent out 97 urine specimens of patients who reported UTI symptoms. Not all were diagnosed with IC, but all showed in the standard office lab tests an indication of infection as, red cells (blood), white cells, and even nitrites.

Results – 3 actually were positive for gram negative, (E. coli) a true urinary tract infection.

Normal urine is sterile.

Urine contains fluids, salts, and waste products, but should not have bacteria.

If there is an infection noted by the laboratory specimen, it is usually E. coli.

The wisdom of wiping front to back is true.

Addressing women – our urethras are only an inch to an inch and a half long. Once a bacterium causes a urethritis it is a short journey to the bladder.

If the physician gives you an antibiotic prescription at the same visit as when you produced the urine specimen, this means that there was no culture and sensitivity lab produced results for his treatment plan. The MD is guessing based on the MD wanting to resolve the problem for a patient in distress by "doing something" and that is often based on a patient demand of the physician to "do something."

Office and ER visits for UTI symptoms.

The point is to have the physician's office or ER send the specimen to the laboratory for both a culture and sensitivity (C&S) to identify the organism to be treated and confirm that it is positive for infection. The second part, the sensitivity part, is to determine the best medication for treatment, and this could include a sulfa-based medication and not an antibiotic.

Good standard of medical practice is to prescribe the correct and least powerful medication to treat the UTI. The reason for the use of the important step of C&S is to not have the too often side problems of yeast infections that often show up as vaginal yeast infections or gastrointestinal, diarrhea miseries. The growing problem of the over use of antibiotics is finally being recognized, but in the urology office it often is still the medication treatment of choice. This means that over time, our personal list of antibiotics we can use to fight infection becomes shorter and the strength needed grows greater; the indication of antibiotic resistant problems.

UTI Symptoms – bacteria caused inflammation? Or IC flare (inflammation)

Always be in doubt and always send it out.

In 48 hours, the lab can say whether there is a bacterial reason for your symptoms and in 72 hours (3 days), the list of medications that match the correct treatment will be available. There is a three-day wait for a medication list of choice, and you have to have a relief rescue.

E. coli causes most infections, but also Chlamydia and Mycoplasma, can be detected with special bacterial cultures.

How to lessen the misery can be by the impact of both bacteria meeting a bladder lining that is vulnerable. The important step of a C&S finds out what is going on so the correct treatment can be ordered.

Waiting for 3 days is not easy when you are miserable and need to be at work and drive the children to soccer practice. This is when the rescue needs to be available.

The rescue treatment for a UTI is virtually the same as if you were having an IC flare.

Inflammation caused perhaps by bacteria exploding nitrates and making a thinned bladder lining even more painful.

1.   More fluids – spring water - void more but diluted urine makes for less discomfort.

2.   AZO, Pyridium, Urelle, Proced (Uriced), all name brands and all mild analgesics (mild for pain) and antiseptic.

3.   Baking soda. Teaspoon in water to drink and cup or more in bath water.

4.   Ice pack to the perineum

5.   Return to the blandest diet you can tolerate. I found baked potatoes, mozzarella cheese, and ground meat with string beans was my dinner for five days running.

6.   Pressure off the pelvic area as in no high heels, cushion on the chair, no long car trips, etc.

My goodness, I have written so much. I know how many mistakes I have made, including demanding antibiotics in my desperate days.

Jo

DECEMBER

From: Jan
To: support@icaction.com
Sent: Saturday, Dec 27, at 7:30 AM
Re: Checking in

Hi Jo,

Wishing you a happy holiday and good health in the coming year!

Wanted to let you know I went on a 5-day clinic to the "Stanford Protocol" in San Francisco last month for pelvic floor dysfunction.

The protocol consisted of hours of training in relaxation and learning how to massage muscle trigger points internally and externally.

My home regimen consists of doing specific stretching exercises at least 2-3 times a day to stretch the pelvic floor muscles, massage myself internally through the rectum and vaginal canal 3 times a week, and listen to a relaxation tape (one series has to do with relaxing and the other series has to do with focusing on certain areas of the body to learn how to relax any tension.) I have a vaginal wand that helps me get the deep internal muscles. Inside, it felt like a hard bone but gradually those ligaments are softening up to feel like real tissue. Intercourse has been extremely painful for me with feelings like a scrub brush around my vagina, and severe pain on the left, where my muscles were so tight. Now I feel some pressure on the left where the muscles are still tighter than normal but intercourse is now enjoyable without pain.

I am happy to have found some thing that is giving me good results.

I am still on Elmiron and plan to stay on it until I can relax the muscles inside more on the left side. I have been able to eat and drink anything lately without any problems.

I guess the most important thing for me is that I have some tools to work with and do not feel panicked when I have increased symptoms. I am grateful to be able to afford the training (very expensive.)

I am also grateful I had your help in the very beginning of my symptoms and was able to stabilize; now hopefully I can help my body to heal even more.

How are things going for you? Jan C.

From: support@icaction.com
To: Jan
Sent: Sunday, Dec 28, at 11:25 AM
Re: <u>Good to hear from you and that you are doing well.</u>

Note: Diagnosed in Feb this year – 11 months to trusting her bladder not to hurt.

Jan:

You are getting to the end of a year of many changes, and I am impressed with how far you have come in a relatively short time. Good work, hard work, well done.

The internal pelvic floor massages for muscle spasms are a success when they are done with trust, care, and expertise. Is there any follow up for the Stanford contact to check that your technique is achieving all it can do?

As you wrote the zinger is cost. I think the ICA should put greater effort into the education of insurance plans to add physical therapy for pelvic pain. Dr. Davis (Ed) says that men generally have an on/off switch for sex; women have multiple buttons.

When you have relaxed your pelvic floor muscles, there is an intangible element of sexual comfort that builds on success, and several for the buttons are pushed for a positive sexual experience. At the IC Clinic, when a person is sexually active (with or with out a partner), we have noted sexual comfort is the true test of how well a person feels they have the pelvic pain of BPS/IC under control. Pelvic relaxation and confidence have blended.

My words of caution are that the pelvic floor tightness can be symptoms of pelvic distress from one or more sources such as the uterus, endometriosis, the lower GI tract, and/or the bladder.

When the pelvic pain is brought on by the bladder lining inflammation and pain fibers firing, there is an ongoing problem that no amount of massage will cure. It is a joint effort of multiple disciplines.

Taking care of your health has served you well and the oral medication, primarily Elmiron, has been part of your regimen on a regular basis.

At the 8 to 9-month mark, the ability to dine with joy rather than eat with caution is a thought to be a gauge of how well your bladder lining is coated. This translates to the pelvic floor responding positively to your massage.

You wrote that you have a rescue package that has grown with options. This translates to the IC symptom bumps that will continue to happen because your life is as active as ever. To me this indicates that Elmiron should not be dismissed. A date would be this coming February to evaluate your oral medication. This opinion is based on both personal and multiple interviews of how comfort and stability can leave our lives when we dismiss medication because we are feeling well.

Examples: In our IC Clinic this past week, I spoke to two women who were there for a yearly checkup. Both reported low bladder/pelvic pain levels of 1 to 2 that translate to the use of the description of "discomfort" only grade of pelvic pain.

Both women wondered with the rising cost of Elmiron and the greatly increased insurance deductible cost if they could cancel or reduce the amount of Elmiron? Both were taking the standard oral dose of 3 capsules per day and both reported the infrequent missed doses that happen because we are human.

With the review of their IC questionnaires, one woman obviously had more of a roller coaster ride of pelvic pain, rising at times of family stress. She was advised to stay on her original medication regimen.

The other women's questionnaires showed she held steady when her pain level was tracked and the changes were in the 1 to 2 discomfort levels. The largest deciding factor - She watched her diet with much more diligence. She is now trying Elmiron 1 capsule on Monday in the AM and 1 capsule in the PM to equal 2 per day as a test. Tuesday 3 capsule, Wednesday 2, etc. to see if she can maintain her pelvic comfort level.

Once again this proves that each of us brings our uniqueness to life and health.

Received an email from a young woman named Brenda. She lives on the East Coast. Her message was - she has been under IC treatment for a year and continues to be in pain. Would you consider communicating with her? Her short email rings with frustration. Thank you for sharing your progress. Happy New Year.

JO Davis

JUNE the NEXT YEAR

From: Jan
To: support@icaction.com
Sent: Wednesday, Jun 30, at 6:57 AM
Re: Status

Hi Jo,

Just to catch you up to date on my progress, I was doing amazingly well on the Elmiron this past year. I was able to eat anything, drink a cup of tea once or twice a day, and have a glass of wine once in a while. I had gotten myself off the Detrol LA and dropped the Prelief pills to cut the acid. Physically, I was able to play basketball with my son, take hikes, and do some minor jogging.

This past month I did myself in during the end of school stress. I was drinking too much tea and when school finished, got off my regular routine of maintenance Elmiron of 2 pills in the morning. I was still trying to take them every other day but got off the regular time and didn't always get the weekends.

So I am now at the beginning of the worst flare I have had since this journey all began and feeling so much remorse for not doing a better job.

I know that I can use all the tools you gave me and I will get better again, so I am not feeling the fear like the first time.

Symptoms are pressure and aching.

I am not sure how to write my summary now. Two months ago it would have been a different story.

Jan

From: support@icaction.com
To: Jan
Sent: Wednesday, Jun 30, 6:19:29 PM
Re: Lesson Learned

Jan:

Learning and learning again is a very human condition.

You know how to make your pelvic area settle down and you are wiser because now you know the choices that got you here and the choices that will calm the flare. It is maddening but you will do it.

That is why I ask you to share your status thoughts - that is real life and more valuable than all the "all is well" messages.

On the list of what you think is the basis of this flare you just addressed; it is a cautionary tale, but let's face it, we all push and do not think about the repercussions. And you sidestepped some of your greatest insurance resources.

Can tell you that after 10 years of hearing Elmiron antidotes, the medication does offer a strong measure of insurance. Not perfect but better than going bare.

What are you doing to make your body happy again?

JO

From: Jan
To: support@icaction.com
Sent: Wednesday, Jun 30, 8:34 PM
Re: Lesson Learned

JO,

In response to this flare, so far I have:

1. Started a food journal again and am writing down what I eat and my body response (usually have pressure feeling an aching in upper thigh area if food triggers me)
2. Went back on 3 Elmiron a day spaced out
3. Started taking Detrol LA for spasms (it really dries me out and makes my voice hoarse) – any suggestions?
4. Stretch 3x per day (suggested Stanford Protocol stretches) and in the morning doing the internal vaginal massage on the left

side where the tight muscles are pulling (have that nasty pain in my left buttock again)

5. Taking Tylenol PM to sleep
6. Using ice after a SHORT walks and stretching. Will try some moderate yoga when feeling a little better - trying to rest a lot and definitely no long walks or jogging.
7. Getting a massage twice a month with someone I worked with before (he focuses on the gluteus and piriformis muscles besides overall)
8. Informing my husband about the flare.
9. Stocking up on no acid organic foods
10. Taking Prelief (over the counter acid relief) before I eat - seemed to help last time
11. Telling myself that I know how to get through this!

JULY

From: Jan
To: support@icaction.com
Sent: Thursday, Jul 01, 10:07 AM
Re: Biotene for dry mouth

Jan:

Your "I'm Doing" list is a good one

Please add lots of spring water – voiding goes up but it is summer and medications like Detrol LA dry us out while they are reducing the feeling of pressure in our bladders.

Are you able to sleep through the night?

Dry mouth – can suggest Biotene and over the counter to respond to mouth dryness,

Salvia protects our teeth and gums. There are other brands but I am familiar with Biotene. It is made in gum, mouthwash, and toothpaste form. And a pocket-sized spray.

Suggest take a fingertip of the Biotene toothpaste and put it in your cheek before bedtime. This helps with the mouth dryness all night.

And yes, you will pull out of this flare.

JO

From: Jan
To: support@icaction.com
Sent: Monday, Jul 05, 10:22 PM
Re: **Need some advice**

In dealing with this latest flare, I added back Detrol LA 1x per day and ½ tab Tylenol PM for sleeping. What is concerning me is now my IBS (Irritable Bowel Syndrome), which developed this past year, is getting worse (pain and stools of different color than usual but not dark as with blood.

I didn't have IBS before when I started Detrol LA so this is a new question. And could the Tylenol also be a factor?

I noticed in one of your emails from our past communications that you mentioned the Detrol LA as needed. How crucial is it if it is affecting the IBS?

Jan

From: support@icaction.com
To: Jan
Sent: Tuesday, Jul 06, 5:00 PM
Re: **My opinion about bowl problems and anticholinergic**

Jan:

Yes, in my opinion a cycle of constipation and/or diarrhea can be brought on by a medication like Detrol.

Classic IBS is a mix of a cycle of constipation and then diarrhea.

The diarrhea may be set off when the hyperactivity of the bowel becomes overwhelming after the irritation of a constipation phase.

Overactive bladder (urgency & frequency) that is a symptom of IC has for symptom control medication like tolterdine (Detrol). It is an anticholinergic that means on the plus side it relaxes the bladder muscle so that the resting pressure in the bladder tolerates more urine collection and the urge to void is lessened.

On the down side is a list of physical complaints beginning with dry mouth, perpetual thirst, and constipation.

This drying affect of an anticholinergic leads to a need for a moistening agent like the over the counter product Biotene to protect your teeth and gums for decay and gum problems. Also needed is a stool softener or a mild laxative for constipation because of the drying action and the lack of muscle activity of the intestines.

The other negative is that with constipation comes bloating and pushing to have bowel movement, not a great situation for a bladder that does not tolerate be pressed upon or pushed around.

What I have found is patients reporting that voiding is more difficult and even had the need to be catheterized in a bladder flare when Detrol, as an anticholinergic example, was added for symptom control. The bladder muscle receives mixed signals because of the inflammation caused spasm and the sphincter muscle does not respond to allow for voiding because of the anticholinergic effect the medication.   I am presuming a cycle of constipation and then diarrhea, I maybe wrong with understanding your situation.

Jo

From: Jan
To: support@icaction.com
Sent: Wednesday, July 7, 7:59:18 AM
Re: Reply for Jan

Hi Jo:

Thank you for your reply.

To answer you question about IBS, my cycle tends more toward diarrhea.

So I guess my question is, if I can't use the Detrol to control bladder spasms, what else can I try? I am wondering if the baking soda/water would be helpful as needed, besides the diet.

Jan

From: support@icaction.com
To: Jan
Sent: Tuesday, July 20, 7:41 PM
Re: hoping rescue regimen worked?

Jan:

Have been out of town – may be too late to answer your question about a homeopathic symptom control for a spastic bladder. Sipping on water that has baking soda mix in can be very helpful. An example would be bottled spring water like Crystal Geyser and a teaspoon of baking soda added to increase the pH.

Two GI stabilization ideas.

The Activia brand yogurt – I have been eating it as my evening desert because it tastes better than my usual plain yogurt. Both greatly lessened the number of diarrhea episodes. Both helped me. But I do not appear to have a lactose sensitivity problem.

Also a good friend who is dealing with post colon surgery has passed on the recommendation form her surgeon to use the product Align.

Summer is escaping.

JO

From: Jan
To: support@icaction.com
Sent: Tuesday, July 20, 9:29 PM
Re: hoping rescue regimen worked?

Hi Jo:

Got quiet for a while because I was trying to figure out how to help the IBS flare I was having. I found a book on line by Heather Van Vorous, "The First Year IBS Irritable Bowel Syndrome" Her message is that you need to always eat soluble fiber first to calm the gut, and then you can eat small amounts of insoluble foods (certain grains, veggies, and fruits.) She also recommended taking Acacia powder to help with either diarrhea or constipation. I was able to slow down the spasm I was having with this diet ad seem to be improving. I think you were right. I had mistakenly thought that high fiber was the best way to help the IBS.

My IC flare is healing. I am able to walk some and eat some foods that used to bother me the first time I had a flare. Things are looking up. Phew!

I did have an annual visit to the urologist last week. He never did tell me if I had blood in my urine and was not interested in setting up an IC support group. "Too much work." He recommended I take Elmiron for 1 month with 2 pills in the morning and 2 pills at night. Then the second month, drop 1 of the pills. Then the third month gets back to maintenance of the 1 in the morning and 1 at night. He mentioned a gel I could use on my arm instead of Detrol LA because it has fewer side effects (dry mouth)

Does this fit in with what your clinic recommends.

What is Align?

Jan

From: Jan
To: support@icaction.com
Sent: Wednesday, July 21, 8:07 AM
Re: Tylenol PM

Hi Jo:

Just wanted to ask if you know if Tylenol PM is a problem or an irritant for people with IBS? From all the Internet info, it does not seem to cause irritation of the gastrointestinal tract.

I have found that it really helps me sleep. But want to make sure I am not causing more irritation for the IBS.

Jan

From: support@icaction.com
To: Jan
Sent: Thursday, July 22, 1:43 PM
Re: Align – Gelnique, Tylenol PM, Elmiron – What I know

Jan:

I want to hug you for being so focused on moving through a lumpy part of the flare. Reread your "care list" and it makes so much sense. You must be the best teacher ever because you follow your own advice.

In response to you last emails the treatment plan using Elmiron is a good one.

Elmiron – In our office most women with a pain level 4 or above are on four (4) Elmiron, 100mg per capsule, per day. – Two (2) in the morning and two (2) in the evening.

I may have written this before but if you have any stomach problems including intestinal issues please do take the medication with some food. The instructions of not eating food one hour before you eat or two hours post food was never FDA tested – it is the default setting for all medication because it was never looked into.

Also I want to add in that with any GI discomfort or upset try removing the medication from the capsule(s) - pull it apart and sprinkle the contents on a teaspoon of apple cause. The protein capsule has been reported to digestive problems for those who are sensitive. Just wondering if your IBS symptoms may be the covering of the capsule?

Three (3) Elmiron per day is the FDA standard but we have found over these many years, that dealing with IC, an extra capsule helps. Maybe it is because if we forget one dose we have at least the 200mg in two (2) for the day.

One point is not to rush to the two (2) capsules a day level unless you think your body has settled into the healing pattern you can trust. You recognize the negative signs. My concern is as you gear up for school on both the family and professional side you body will be demanding more care.

Align - is a Probiotic. What is a probiotic?

Probiotic: A microbe that protects its host and prevents disease. Generally speaking probiotic products can help restore normal balance of intestinal bacteria.

In the Align product, the active microbe is known as B.ifantis. The best-known probiotic is Lactobacillus acidophilus, which is found in yogurt, acidophilus milk, and supplements. Probiotics counter the decimation of helpful intestinal bacterial by antibiotics. Probiotics given in combination with antibiotics are useful in preventing antibiotic-associated diarrhea. The yeast S. boulardii and three strains of lactobacillus have been shown to be useful in this regard.

Align in the ivory green box has no soy meaning no MSG.

Made from milk protein – casemate – lactose free

No gelatin

No Dietary fiber

Writing on capsule does have artificial color – FD & C blue

More information on the web

Another brand that is often recommended by physicians is Lactinex. This product contains the bacteria Lactobacillus acidophilus.

Probiotics have also been used for the restoration of needed bacteria in the vagina destroyed with the use of antibiotics.

Gelnique - I think that is topical application of the medication what you are referring to when you wrote that your Urologist gave you a topical gel for over active bladder symptoms?

Gelnique by Watson, Inc. was FDA approved in 2009 and has as its active ingredient Oxybutynin chloride (an anticholinergic). This chemical has been the basis of multiple OAB symptom control products.

Inactive ingredients in Gelnique are alcohol, USP, glycerin, USP: hydroxypropyl cellulose, NF; sodium hydroxide, NF; and purified water, USP.

Gelnique active anticholinergic agent is no different from any oxybutynin product – what is different is the method of administration and that can make all the difference in reducing the negative affects of dry mouth, constipation, etc.

Gelnique, a topical gel, when applied to the skin means it medication does not go through the digestive track and then to the liver, our bodies' major filtering system, in its strongest form; but through the skin in the blood system in a smaller and more measured amounts. The filtering through the liver on the first go around is not as potent and so the drying effects (this is what anticholinergics do – dry out cells as well as other chemically caused effects such as possible rapid heartbeat.) are less and so the annoying effects are less.

For you the question: Is the reduction of the urge and frequency symptoms using the gel producing any greater bladder pain or compromising your ability to void?

Tylenol PM is one of my favorites for pain control because the touch of the Benadryl makes it a combination of an antihistamine to help reduce mast cell activity caused by allergies. Perhaps even the bladder inflammation is reduced and also the side affect of sleep inducing at night is helpful. And it has no ephedrine that causes bladder problems. Hope this helps.

JO

From: Jan
To: support@icaction.com
Sent: Friday, July 23, 7:24:31 AM
Re: Align – Gelnique, Tylenol PM, Elmiron – Great Info

Hi, Jo

Thank you for all the great info and lists of ingredients. You have an amazing library of knowledge.

And thank you for the complement!

I actually yelled out loud with happiness when I read that you do not need to worry so much about the timing of taking the Elmiron around food. That has been such a difficult thing for me; to time with my schedule and be able to eat several times a day which I prefer to 3 times a day when on Elmiron. That was huge news for me.

I am not clear if the Tylenol PM can irritate the GI tract (small and large intestines). Most of the internet info says no.

I really do need to sleep better but am very hesitant to take anything that could irritate any part of my colon. Last year I had atypical ulcers and I think it may have just had the same thing with some of my IBS symptoms

Do you have any other info on the Tylenol PM effect on the colon?

Jan

From: Jan
To: support@icaction.com
Sent: Sunday, July 25, 9:06 AM
Re: Address for IC Clinic

Hi JO:

I hope you realize the difference you are making in many people's lives. You have made such a positive impact on my journey, and I am so happy to be able to give back to help out other women who are finding themselves on the same journey.

I think it is very important that in my follow-up note that I stress the need to stay on Elmiron. The Stanford Clinic gave me the hope that I might just be reacting to stress with pelvic tightening, but now I think it stems from my bladder.

Continuing to work on my present flare. I am able to deal with the ups and downs with some confidence these days.

Jan

From: Jan
To: support@icaction.com
Sent: Tuesday, July 27, 4:00 PM
Re: **Elmiron side effects**

Hi Jo:

I have to ask you about the side effects of Elmiron. I have been having IBS diarrhea for the last year with one incident of blood in my stools. The doctor did a colonoscopy and saw atypical ulcers in my colon that were starting to heal.

The last couple of weeks, I have been having blood in my stool even though I have been on a low acid IC diet.

When I looked up Elmiron side effects today, it mentioned diarrhea and blood in the stool as a possible side effect in 1 percent to 4 percent of people who used it.

What can you tell me about this?

I am going to my primary doctor tomorrow to get a referral back to the gastroenterologist I saw a year ago. I hope I can get in quickly.

I may need to try a break from the Elmiron, which worries me.

Jan

From: support@icaction.com
To: Jan
Sent: Tuesday, July 27, 5:37 PM
Re: **Elmiron side effects – complete email**

Post-marketing Experience

From Elmiron Web site

Rectal Hemorrhage: Information from Ortho-McNeil web site

ELMIRON was evaluated in a random, double blind, parallel group. Phase 4 study conducted in 380 patients with interstitial cystitis dosed for 32 weeks. At a daily dose of 300mg (n=128), rectal hemorrhage was reported as an adverse event in 6.3% of patients. The severity of the events was described as "mild" in most patients. Patients in that study who were administered ELMIRON 900 mg daily, a dose higher than the approved (FDA) dose, experienced a higher incidence of rectal hemorrhage, 15%.

To me this means that as a heparin like (weak but there all the same) product it can cause GI bleeding as the dose increased (described as higher than approved) number of incidences went up. If my math is correct in a group of 380 – 16 patients would have had rectal bleeding.

www.OrthoMcNeil.com asks for adverse events to be reported. They have an on going database of observations. Elmiron has been FDA approved since 1996 so there is quite a track record.

As a side note, Elmiron has been proven to pass through the GI track without absorption. In the urine, it has about a 1-3% amount that stays behind and is thought to make up the barrier to help the damaged epithelium layer of the bladder push away the caustic urine and by doing so it is thought the nerve fibers/pain fibers <u>do not</u> begin cause a PBS/IC flare.

If you bruise easily and are on any anticoagulant like substance, even fish oil and a baby aspirin day, this should be shared with your urologist and GI M.D. You asked about acetaminophen (Tylenol) and liver enzymes going up – there is a small chance combined with Elmiron – tolerance is less and prothrombin time can be affected. Again the confusion starts with how much is too much for each individual.

With your past GI symptoms, your Gastroenterologist (GI) and Urologist need to be informed of the rectal bleeding.

This is my long-winded way of saying, I would find out why these symptoms are occurring. Rectal bleeding may be one reason to consider direct bladder instillations and by pass the body's general circulation.

When there is a flare it does make for a renewed appreciation for spring water, baked potatoes, rice, and ice packs as important adjuncts to healing.

I just asked Ed and he said "tell your physicians all your symptoms."

Please tell me what is going on.

JO

From: Jan
To: support@icaction.com
Sent: Thursday, July 29, 7:30:13 AM
Re: Latest developments

Hi, Jo:

I still do not have a definite idea about what is been causing the blood in my stools.

I saw my primary physician to get a referral to my urologist to hopefully get me in sooner. She did a brief rectal exam and did see some inflammation in some internal hemorrhoids.

The urologist assistant I saw yesterday did not know about blood in the stool being a possible side effect (Elmiron). She advised that I stay off the Elmiron until the urologist can check me. So she gave me a prescription for Gelnique (for bladder control) and amitriptyline (Elavil) for pain. I am sticking to a bland soft food diet, mild exercise with ice packs and stretching, and lots of water.

I have an appointment in 6 weeks for follow-up with the urologist.

The diet has pretty much slowed down the diarrhea, so if it is hemorrhoids, there should be improvement.

Hope this blows over quickly so I can get back to the Elmiron treatment.

Jan

AUGUST

From: Jan
To: support@icaction.com
Sent: Sunday, August 1, 9:02:29 AM
Re: Mail

Hi, Jo:

I loved your latest emails......thanks!

When I met with the urologist's assistant this past week, I did tell her about your clinic and gave her your email address to contact. She was interested in the booklet you are publishing since many patients in this area are looking for support. Jan

SEPTEMBER

From: Jan
To: support@icaction.com
Sent: Thursday, September 16, 5:58 AM
Re: Update and question

Hi Jo:

How are things going?

I have been healing from the flare I had at the end of school.

I did go back on the Elmiron after checking in with the urologist.

Between the Elmiron and a strict bland diet, my IC healed quickly.

The irritable bowel has been longer in healing but I made a lot of progress. I had been having urges to have a BM as soon as food entered my mouth.

I have been able to slow down my system with the bland diet. I am also listening to stress reduction tapes daily.

What I am curious to find out about from your clinic is this: Are there links between IC and having small ulcers in you colon?

My gastroenterologist scoped my lower colon and found a few atypical ulcers.

I have fewer than when he saw me last Christmas when I also had another flare.

I would appreciate any medical info you have on this. Have not been able to find any information on line.

Thanks!

Jan

From: support@icaction.com
To: Jan
Sent: Thursday, September 16, 3:50:56 P
Re: Update and question

Hello Jan:
It must be email telepathy to hear from you.

About you ulcer question –

Time magazine at least 4 years ago had an in-depth front cover/feature about inflammation and pointed to it as the basis for most of our chronic ills, including hypertension, ulcers, cancer, etc.

The first time I heard inflammation discussed was at least 8 years ago at a lecture given by an MD/Professor from the UN. of Oklahoma. He was a speaker at an IC conference; Dr. Miner was his last name. His point was that IC was connected to other inflammation conditions. The "mast" cells that are part of our natural protective system over react.

As time has pasted studies show that IC, IBS, migraine headaches, Fibromyalgia are all inflammation based.

Simplistically, that would mean that there is increased inflammation in part of the body as the major focus but also inflammation could show up in other forms and to a lesser degree – colon ulcerations.

Question is what brings on the inflammation? That is the body's protective mechanism that goes on over drive with activity and then you have allergy symptoms for example.

The mast cell does its job too well and releases histamine and inflammation is the result. Inflammation is swelling- swelling presses on nerve fibers equaling pain or the urge to void or evacuate your bowels.

Think a source of information would be to research inflammation and see if you make a personal connection.

JO

Received by mail from Jan:

2 August

"What I think - the past two years"

Here is a list of what I think after a couple of years dealing with IC. My urologist was open to prescribing physical therapy (internal and external massage) to help me with muscle tension

1. It was very important to me to find an urologist who had a positive attitude that I could manage IC and live a good life.

2. At first I was very depressed in reading other IC patients stories online. When I redirected my energy to finding all the resources or tools to deal with the condition I started feeling more encouraged and optimistic.

3. Finding a support person online was huge in my ability to keep trying to improve my condition. There is no local support group in my hometown.

4. I not only tried the IC diet, slowing down on my exercise, icing and stretching, but learned how to relax my pelvic area muscles with massage. I was trained in relaxation and internal and external massage in a workshop in San Francisco. It was very expensive, but really helped with the aching in my pelvic area and pain with intercourse. I have also been able to stop feelings of pressure in the anal area, and a constant feeling of having to use the bathroom.

5. I continue to work on becoming more relaxed in my daily interactions. I have always been a high anxiety person and am learning through yoga, relaxation tapes, and focusing on the positive moments throughout my day to reduce my negative thing tendencies. I am aware that so much of my tension is stored in the pelvic area.

6. It is easy to become totally caught up at first in learning how to mange the IC symptoms. After starting the Elmiron, diet, and massage, and seeing huge improvement in 6 months, I was able to relax and move back towards the things I enjoy.

7. I have learned that once you have stabilized, you have to remember to keep taking Elmiron and stick to the diet. I have

had some flares during times of stress when I have gotten somewhat careless in following the diet and sticking to the medication regimen.

8. My family and friends have gone through the ups and down with me, it has been sad at times to restrict or modify my activities with them, but I have had to listen to my body and treat it with care. As my bladder improved with all my self care tools and medications, I was able to start getting back to participating

9. I continue to have some ups and downs, but have seen such an improvement in the 2 years since I have been diagnosed. It is encouraging to see the progress and know that life can be good.

10. These thoughts have become helpful reminders to me on what to focus on: "Faith is trusting in the good. Fear is putting your trust in the bad."

19. Ana, age 69
Mal de Orin

Background

My name is Ana, and I am 69 yrs. old. I was born in San Salvador, El Salvador, Central America. I came to the USA when I was 20 yrs. old. At that time, I did not have any IC problems. My IC symptoms, which have consisted of pain when voiding, feelings that my pelvic area is on fire, frequent bathroom visits and/or urgency, have been intermittent since the late "60's. There have been periods when I have been "symptom free". However, looking back I recall that as a young child I did have occasional bouts of burning sensation when I urinated and numerous trips to the bathroom to void as if I had a full bladder.

My mother was a single parent and she had to work long hours, therefore, different babysitters cared me for during my growing up years until I was placed in a boarding school. When I occasionally complained of burning sensation or repeated visits to the bathroom, I was advised to either sit in warm water or put salt on my navel. Sometimes I was told that my symptoms were brought on either because I had sat on something cold or something hot, i.e., tile or cement.

It should be noted that in the process of writing this paper I asked 6 different female friends from El Salvador what they had heard, when they were young, was the cause of the "**Mal de Orin**" (**Mal de Orin** refers to the burning, frequency and urgency symptoms). Their responses were the same: Not to sit on something hot or they would get "Mal de Orin".

When asked what they had heard as to how to treat the **"Mal de Orin"**, their responses were: sit in warm water, put salt in your navel, drink lots of water, drink water mixed with sugar and salt or drink Tamarind Water – This is a dried fruit that is sold in the Salvadorian and Mexican markets and people drink it instead of a soda at home or in a restaurant. It is a refreshing drink.

Back to my personal history - since my IC saga began (late 60's), during a "flare up" I would go to the urologist. In those days the form of treatment was a very painful procedure that is called Urethra Dilatation, which consisted of cutting scar tissue from the urethra with a surgical metal rod. I would also be given a prescription for Pyridium which made the color of my urine orange. I do not remember if I was also given a prescription for antibiotics to prevent an infection after the above procedure. This form of treatment went on for a few years. Although I did respond to the treatment within a short time, it was not the appropriate modality, but that was the form of intervention that was recommended at that time.

In fact, I was appalled to have learned recently that Urethra Dilatation continues to be used by some doctors even though it is a very painful experience and presently there are better diagnostic and treatment modalities.

In the fall of 1981, I was admitted to the hospital and had a Urethra Dilatation under anesthesia. My symptoms went into remission for a few years – possibly this was a lucky coincidence though. Furthermore, I did not have any IC symptoms at that time.

I have been very fortunate that my IC symptoms have not included ongoing pelvic pain, which would interfere with sexual intercourse. Pelvic pain is present only when I am in the middle of a flare up. I was also blessed that I was not bothered with IC flare-ups during my pregnancy in 1982.

However, my symptoms returned with a vengeance during the 90's. The flare-ups would occur approximately every 3 or 4 months apart approximately. At that time, I was only treated with antibiotics despite the fact that the lab work was negative for a urinary tract infection. But the symptoms went away. I know that antibiotics are not recommended now.

In desperation and looking for a "cure", I sought a consultation at a teaching hospital for my IC symptoms sometime in the 90's. To my surprise and terror, I was even tested to rule out AIDS. I was filled with anxiety and panic while I waited for approximately 5 weeks, I believe, for the results, which were negative thanks to God. After all the test results were in, to my dismay, the treatment recommendation was the same as the one from my OBYN: use yeast vaginal cream about 3 times a week. This did not help of course.

I then began a pattern of being seen in Urgent Care on a walking basis; the lab work was negative for a UTI, but nevertheless I received a prescription for antibiotics, which offered me almost immediate relief. Going to Urgent Care was convenient because I did not need an appointment and I could go after work, after hours or on weekends as needed. I was well until the next flare up and the cycle would repeat itself again and again.

I continued to have flare ups and I again went for another consultation to another teaching hospital in 2007. The main reason for seeking another consultation was due to the fact that I had now become allergic to 3 antibiotics: Bactrim, Cipro and Keflex. This time I was given the Elmiron IC Smart Diet. At this time, I had no idea what IC stands for or what it is. I was not really told what my diagnosis was or what I had. Medication was briefly discussed as a possibility. However, I decided not to go back because I felt I was not being heard or guided appropriately. Later I requested a copy of the consultation report that documented that if there was no improvement with, "diet modification alone…one thing we need to contemplate is getting her evaluated with an MRI of the pelvis to rule out urethral diverticulum as well."

In looking back, I feel that the IC diet needed to have been discussed and emphasized. The BPS/ IC diet, suggested by the makers of Elmiron, looked so restricted that I thought, "What can I eat then? Forget it. I'm not going back". This was my second reason for not going back.

In January 2009, I was lucky to read in the local newspaper about the IC Support group meeting that is held at the Foothill Presbyterian Hospital in Glendora every other month. I attended my first meeting, which was conducted by Dr. E. Davis and Mrs. Jo Davis, RN. The meeting was so informative that I decided immediately to make an appointment to see Dr. Davis for a consultation.

Dr. Davis confirmed the IC Diagnosis through a procedure, which is done under general anesthesia on an outpatient basis at the Presbyterian hospital. It should be noted that upon my discharge I was also given a very informative piece of paper about Elmiron which stated that Elmiron is, "a protectant used to treat interstitial cystitis."

Further testing was also done at the clinic to establish a treatment plan. After all procedures, i.e., Cystoscopy, urodynamic test and lab work were completed I was placed on Elmiron to treat my IC symptoms. It took a couple of months, I believe, before my bladder calmed down from the very painful flare up that I was going through five years ago.

Where am I now?

At this time, I think that I have learned to manage my IC symptoms to the best of my ability. So far I have not had a flare up since I have been in treatment with Dr. Davis. Unfortunately I had to stop Elmiron in the fall of 2012 because I developed a skin rash. Presently I am able to eat various foods, vegetables and fruit. But, I am still somewhat cautious with acidic foods

Since I discontinued Elmiron, I have used the following: I am taking Marshmallow Root Powder. I take 1 capsule per day. However, this is a lot of work since I have to fill the capsules myself. However, Nature's Way sells the Marshmallow 455 mg capsules already prepared. When I finish the Marshmallow root powder, I may switch to the prepared formula. I have also learned recently that there is Marshmallow Root tea.

In the past, I took Corn Silk capsules 450 mg, which you can buy at the Vitamin Shoppe.

I only took 1 a day; they also have the Tea, which I have not tried yet. I am postponing taking any teas at this time because I don't need it.

So far I do not drink any coffee, tea or sodas and rarely eat spicy food, but I have been eating all kind of fruits - not strawberries, mangos, citrus or any kind of melons. I know that spicy food and fruit affect me so I take Prelief to decrease the acidity in the food when I eat them. I do not recommend this though. Diet is very important. However, during my last visit to the Urologist the Physician Asst., instructed me to watch my diet closely and not to eat all the forbidden foods to prevent a flare up – which I definitely do not want!

During the summer, I swim every day and I know that the chlorine sometimes bothers my bladder so when I have IC symptoms, I use a vaginal cream only in the affected area. This cream calms down my symptoms after a few minutes.

My 30 yrs. old daughter lived in Germany for about 7 years and while living there she began to suffer IC symptoms, which I believe, were treated as yeast infections or urinary tract infections. She returned to the USA in the fall of 2009. Occasionally, I shared with her some of the IC symptoms I was having, the medical treatment I was receiving, the medication I was taking, the IC Clinic appointments and IC Support meetings that I was attending plus the relief I was getting. To my surprise, she then admitted that she was experiencing some of the discomfort that I experienced prior to taking Elmiron.

My daughter is a vegetarian so she is against taking capsules because according to her they are made of some animal's parts. She also is against taking any type of medications. At the time of this writing, she has not sought any medical intervention because she now knows that BPS/IC is a chronic disease and that would have labeled her as having a pre-existing condition, which would disqualify her for medical insurance coverage.

While living in Germany, my daughter's primary doctor would initially recommend that she try first a natural product rather than prescribe a regular medication. Therefore, when she learned about IC, she did some research and decided to use the following:

Marshmallow Root drops 450 mg. alcohol free (1 Oz costs $11.00+. She fills the dropper or takes only 2/3 of it, depending on the level of her symptoms, in a small amount of water. I have not tried the drops because they are too expensive, but they work for her.

These drops calm down her IC symptoms (whatever they might be), but she does not watch her diet. She eats hot peppers and hot sauce plus spicy and acidic foods on a daily basis, which I don't recommend.

Unfortunately, My 50 year old niece just began to have urgency and some pelvic pressure problems a few months ago. She works on a telecommute position, but most of the time she spends it at home sitting in front of the computer doing her job. She has now been placed on Amitriptyline to resolve her discomfort. So far she is responding well and I wish her the best.

What I think helped me to manage my IC symptoms?

1. Seeking treatment with a board certified urologist whose practice includes treating patients with a diagnosis of IC. Because IC is a chronic disease, it has been very important for me to keep my appointments, listen closely to the wealth of information that has been provided to me by the staff of the IC team and take notes for future reference.

2. Finding a doctor that listened to my personal story and understood the description of my individual symptoms was a relief in itself. I have never felt that my urologist dismissed any of my questions or personal concerns.

3. I have learned firsthand how to best treat my individual symptoms in a very supportive environment through the IC team staff. And, when I feel that I am beginning to experience some discomfort because of something that I ate or drank I proceed to implement something that I have learned. For example, I know that spicy food, some fruits and some teas will cause me burning and painful symptoms. When I know that I will eat/drink any of the above I take Prelief to take the acid out of the food. If symptoms develop, I soak myself in a warm tub with baking soda, use a cold pack and the next day I am well. Occasionally, if all of a sudden, I wake up in the morning with a burning sensation, I apply externally Estrace (Estradiol), which is a vaginal cream. However, what I really need to learn is to stay away from any potential offenders. I need to keep in mind that the food stays in my mouth only for few "seconds", but the symptoms could lead to a "flare up". Definitely I need to continue to work on my IC diet.

4. By attending the IC Support Group, I gained an understanding what IC is. I was then able to share some of the information with my family members. I felt validated that I had a "real" and not an "imaginary" condition. In sharing this information, my daughter discovered that she has the same condition. My daughter is attempting to treat her symptoms on her own and is waiting to change her health insurance at the appropriate time. Also, my niece disclosed that she was having some similar symptoms. I encouraged her to go to her doctor and she is now in treatment.

5. Recently I realized that when I am out with family members I visit the ladies room more frequently that when I am out with friends. This is something that I will now have to work on. I have now also noticed that I use the bathroom more often when I am at home than when I am out. Perhaps I will now try to work on bladder training by letting longer periods of time pass before voiding.

6. I was meditating for 20 minutes on a daily basis to decrease the stress of the day, but recently I have not been doing it. I need to continue on a regular basis. I view the above as a preventive practice since stress can increase the intensity of any IC symptoms.

7. I read an article in my local paper by Sue Manning (Associate Press) that according to an Ohio State University study, "Healthy cats show sign of illness when stressed. At the same time, cats diagnosed with feline interstitial cystitis, or FIC, became healthier when stress levels were reduced, the study show."

8. I learned through my own personal experience that some medical staff still does not know how to treat IC. In the past, I was encouraged to drink plenty of cranberry juice. Now I know that "cranberry juice" is not meant for the person who has IC due to its high acidic content. In the past, I drank cranberry juice before I left home for a social activity as a "preventive measure" and to protect my bladder. It took me sometime to realize that "cranberry juice" was bringing on symptoms of an overactive bladder. Cranberry juice: most of the standard brands are more water and sugar than cranberries. The cranberry pills however are heavy with vitamin C as the main ingredient. I found out that one of my triggers was acid and whether it was an orange, Vitamin C, or dark green vegetables I should watch my choices.

9. I wish you well in your search for the best path to follow to have your IC symptoms become manageable. I know the stress that comes with wanting an answer to how to deal with the pelvic pain and its wandering ways. My advice is to give yourself the gift of allowing for errors that happen in the choices you make. And when the good moments come ask what made this minute, hour, day, better – Sometimes it is a good night's sleep, sometimes it is TV novella, often it is a warm bath with baking soda.

10. Find support – Someone to talk to.

20. Kristin, age 25
My Extraordinary Journey with Bladder Pain Syndrome

Background

Kristin tells her BPS/IC story with all the twists and turns that have made so many of us wonder who we can trust. She took her questions, searched and found answers.

Kristin's Story

Have you ever felt symptoms of a urinary tract infection, but doctors constantly insist you don't have one? If you answered yes to this question, as I did at the age of nineteen, you may be a prime candidate for a commonly misdiagnosed or missed bladder disorder called Interstitial Cystitis or Bladder Pain Syndrome. My life before chronic bladder infection symptoms was happy and full of fun memories. I grew up in Orange County, California and was a healthy, active, young lady who was heavily involved in various school functions and church. I had always felt the urge to urinate more frequent than any other of my friends and continually felt like I had a urinary tract infection. Unfortunately, detecting this disease can be extremely hard because its symptoms are identical to a traditional bladder infection and often are fused with what seems to be menstrual pain. In the fall of 2008, I had two exams, a laparoscopy and cystoscopy; this is when my pelvic pain issues were labeled the "evil twins" by the gynecologic and urologist; I had drawn the genetic ticket saying Endometriosis and Interstitial Cystitis. At the age of nineteen, I had a diagnoses of defective bladder lining (IC) and uterine cells that are outside the uterus (Endo); both consequently cost three painful years of my life and an extraordinary journey I will never soon forget.

The Beginning of my Endeavor:

My journey began in late fall about six years ago, when I started suffering from what seemed to be a reoccurring bladder infection. I would feel a constant urge to urinate even after I had already used the restroom, pressure on my bladder and lower abdomen, and a burning sensation after urinating. I would have to use the restroom at least 25 times a day and about 4 times a night. I was visiting my local doctor's office about two times a month, complaining of severe bladder discomfort and pain. Whenever the doctors would hear about my symptoms, they would immediately give me a urine test to check for a urinary tract infection. The interesting thing was that all of my test results would come back negative for a bladder infection. Even though there was no evidence of an infection, the doctors would persistently prescribe antibiotics. I never quite understood why they did this, but I trusted their judgment and would take the medication. They explained that some women and men were just more prone to urinary tract infections and that I should not be concerned at all. After continuing this tedious routine for approximately three years, I had finally suffered enough and decided to consult a specialist in urology. What I did not realize was that this was going to be the wisest decision I could have ever made.

The Doctor that Changed my Life:

I knew that I wanted to see a specialist in my local area, so I researched online and found a doctor in Glendora who under stood BPS/IC. He had great reviews and was only about 20 minutes away from my house. I decided to make an appointment so that I could hopefully get an explanation for what I had been experiencing.

When I finally met up with Dr. Davis, I explained my story and told him what the other doctors had done to try to help me. He was not surprised but discouraged to hear that doctors actually gave me antibiotics for an infection that I never had. He then looked at me and said two words that changed my life forever. He told me that I most likely had a very common bladder disorder called Bladder Pain Syndrome (BPS) Interstitial Cystitis (IC). BPS/IC is a chronic condition consisting of pelvic pain, pressure, or discomfort in the bladder and pelvic region due to a lack of protective coating around the bladder. Dr. Davis told me that in order to determine if I truly had BPS/IC, he would have to perform a cystoscopy. A cystoscopy is an outpatient procedure that required to be done when I am under anesthesia; it allows a physician to see the interior surface of the bladder in order to look for signs of the disease. I was in complete shock because I had never heard of this disease, and now I would have to undergo surgery in order to be properly diagnosed.

At this point, I was so sick of living in pain that I immediately agreed to have surgery. A week after my procedure, I met up with Dr. Davis and was told that I indeed had I BPS/IC. I was so relieved that I finally had an answer to my horrible problem, but extremely mad at the same time. How it could be that after three years of going to four different doctors, not one had even suspected that I might have BPS/IC?

Why BPS/IC is Commonly Misdiagnosed:

According to Dr. Davis, one of the main reasons why BPS/IC is so commonly misdiagnosed is that there is no precise diagnostic test that can be given to detect it. The only way it can be accurately detected is through a cystoscopy.

The second reason BPS/IC is so commonly misdiagnosed is that the symptoms of this disorder are nearly identical to the "common" bladder infection. Many doctors misinterpreted the traditional BPS/IC symptoms for a urinary tract infection and ended up prescribing unnecessary medications.

Even though IC is a chronic disorder that will never officially go away, there are medications available to help people manage it. The key is to be properly diagnosed, so that patients can begin receiving help.

What I did once I was diagnosed with IC:

Once I became diagnosed with this disorder, Dr. Davis educated me on different sets of medications that would work for my body to properly help me cope with this chronic illness. I was put on a drug called Elmiron to help build a protective coating around my bladder. They also gave me a low dose of an antidepressant called Amitriptyline to relieve some of the pain and to help calm the nerve endings around my bladder. I also take an antihistamine to reduce inflammation and swelling. This set of medications works very well for me, but everyone is different and it is key to work with your doctor to see what set of medications work well for you. On days when I have a flare up, I drink lots of water and take a medication called Uristat (phenazopyrid), which puts a coating around your bladder and temporally numbs the pain and reduce urgency.

The second thing I learned after becoming diagnosed with BPS/IC was how to change my dietary lifestyle. I learned that patients with this disorder are put on a strict diet that helps reduce food irritants from penetrating the bladder. I was also taught how to manage my stress levels, since stress is a major bladder irritant.

The third and most important thing I learned through my whole BPS/IC endeavor is that I was not alone. There are hundreds of thousands of other people who are going through the same thing you are! You are not alone!!!! With that being said, it is very important to have a strong support team at home. I am very fortunate to have a family and a husband who understands what I go through, and they have been there for me since the day I was diagnosed. I found that by being open with my friends and family about my condition, they were better equipped to help me live out my day-to-day life as a normal young woman. For example, when my husband and I go out to dinner, he always looks through the menu with me to help to find something that is appropriate to eat that will not irritate my bladder. Having people that know your condition and all that it entails is paramount for your road to recovery.

Living Life with BPS/IC:

I am now a healthy 25 year old woman, who is married and living every day to its fullest. I have a great job and plan on starting a family in the near future. Since I was diagnosed three years ago, I have been on medications to help decrease my pain and help build a coating around my bladder. Now, I rarely have any symptoms, and I know what to do to help myself on a bad day.

For people that are experiencing similar symptoms, get checked out immediately. I only wish that I had heard about this disorder years ago so that I could have eliminated all the needless pain and suffering. The problem with BPS/IC is that it is so commonly misdiagnosed and people must endure their symptoms much longer than they need to. My goal is to spread the word about this disease in hopes of helping others!

What I Think – The Top 10 things that have helped me cope and live with BPS/IC:

1. Use ice packs or frozen bottles of water in between your legs and above your lower abdomen when you are having a flare.

2. Drink at least 7 glasses of water a day (on top of the other liquids you drink throughout your day). It will help dilute your urine and make it less acidic (especially when you are having a bladder flare!!!)

3. If you are a stressful person, like I am, the use of aromatherapies during showers and before going to bed will help your body relax; which in turn, will let your bladder relax and not be so tense.

4. Stick to a strict BPS/IC diet for the first 6 months after being diagnosed to let the Elmiron do its job. Then, you can slowly work other things into your diet to see how your bladder reacts to them.

5. If Elmiron is too expensive for you, even with insurance; you can print a manufacturer's coupon to help you out for a few months. (Just look up the Elmiron website, and it will walk you through the process on getting a coupon.)

6. I sometimes take Prelief, a pill that you can take with your food/drink to reduce the acidity of the food/drink you ingest (especially if you plan on drinking or eating something that you know may upset your bladder!)

7. By just eliminating one thing from your diet, you may feel a lot better. For example, my bladder does not like coffee. Even if I have followed my diet for weeks, if I drink even one cup of coffee I can have a flare that last days.

8. My bladder is ok with Coke products, but cannot stand any Pepsi products. (Pepsi products contain more potassium then Coke products and my bladder cannot stand potassium.)

9. I like to wear stretchy clothes because constricting pants puts pressure on my lower back and abdomen and exacerbates my bladder flares.

10. My top trigger foods/drinks are: coffee, alcohol, tomato sauce, and chocolate, sour candy, rye bread, bananas and oranges. (If I ever cheat and do consume one of these types of food or drink, I make sure I drink a lot of water to dilute its potency.)

In Conclusion:

What I learned from going through this long, grueling journey was that you should never accept a diagnosis that doesn't make sense. If you feel that you are constantly going back to a doctor with the same symptoms and no success in treatment, perhaps it's time to speak up and ask more questions or look around for someone more specialized in the area of your symptoms. Don't be afraid to research and find a doctor that might have the help you need. I let three years pass by before realizing that I needed to take charge of finding help for myself. If I had not done this, I might still be living in so much pain. You know your body better than anyone else and never forget that! If you want further information on BPS/IC, you can visit www.ichelp.org or call 1-800-HELP-ICA.

Where do I go from here?

At the end of every chapter you have read ten specific items that each writer wanted to share. As we reread each story and reviewed the "What I Think" pages, we like you, noticed that there are connections between the discoveries of how individuals have come to cope with BPS/IC. We picked the following top 20 thoughts we think give the guidance and support that is the spirit of this book.

Top twenty "What I think"

1. *You* have IC; IC <u>does not</u> have you. This is extremely important when dealing with the daily ups and downs of Interstitial Cystitis. Don't let your life come to a halt. Learn how to help yourself and take control of your disease. Do not let your disease control you.

2. Educate yourself. Seek information wherever you can find it. Internet (i.e. ICA, IC Network, icaction.com), medical journals, research, etc. The more you know and soak in, the more you will learn how to live and deal with IC. Remember there are lots of good ideas but not all of them are right for you.

3. Laugh. Have a sense of humor. If you don't have one, get one quick. Laughter has helped us through some tough and painful episodes, awkward situations and stressful times. Make yourself laugh. Finding humor in things that you never found funny or amusing before will be one of your greatest supports though your IC journey.

4. Do not EVER let anyone tell you that the pain is not real. Sexual pain, pain when you go to the bathroom, aching, throbbing, constant pressure pain, etc. The pain is REAL. You have to be willing to do something about it. Whether it is seeking the comfort of an ice pack, heating pad, a warm baking soda bath, taking painkiller, relaxation techniques, etc. Learn how to help yourself and then force yourself to do it. It will be easier the next time because you will know what works.

5. Diet is often the last item that is recognized as an influence in IC, I think it is more than 50% of control of symptoms. Watch your diet. You can ignore what you eat and drink, but eventually it will catch up to you and your bladder. Often the trigger is the food source (try true organic) or how it's prepared, or size or number of servings. Start with removing acidic foods from your diet, that means coffee and tea with the chemical double whammy of caffeine and acid.

6. Keep a food journal. Our support group's website, www.icaction.com, has a 24 hour form that keeps you on track and lists trips to the bathroom and pain level. Change nothing for three days. I found I had one glass of water in the early morning and then no water until lunch; I never realized it until I completed a three day log.

7. Your water source and amount you drink not only dilutes the urine but when water has minerals or "spring' water it's slightly less acidic. Both elements help the damaged bladder lining to heal and control greater inflammation.

8. Don't ignore symptoms – Sexual pain, microscopic blood in your urine, constant bladder infections, don't let the medical community write you off, keep fighting and searching for a doctor with knowledge and one that will listen to your needs, feelings, symptoms, etc. and most importantly, a doctor who will *believe* you.

9. Be prepared to search for a physician who understands IC. This situation of lack of awareness is improving, but there is still a less than perfect system of identification and treatment.

10. If your health care source is not responding to your call for help perhaps you need another opinion. For me antibiotics prescriptions clouded the issue of an inflammatory bladder disease that required specific medications and support.

11. Remember the words exercise, lifting, footwear with support. - For me it is walking and working in my garden – I needed to learn that pain means no gain.

12. Before this IC pain hit I was anti medication. Now I know there are medications I require and I make sure I know why I am taking each one.

13. Made a point of educating myself so the word chronic did not mean the scary unknown.

14. A support group helps to reinforce you are not alone. Find an online friend to share information.

15. Put yourself first. Take time to relax and pamper yourself. Get rid of stress as much as possible and inundate yourself with positive self-talk and surroundings. There are times there is too much on your list of good works and you need to say "not now."

16. Learn relaxation techniques, I know it is easier to say and harder to do, but the feeling of being over whelmed can take all body pain to a higher level. Practice the techniques of quieting your pain demons before pain becomes overwhelming.

17. The Interstitial Cystitis Association (ICA) should be pushing for a test for IC. Physicians rarely think about the connection of bladder/pelvic pain to IC. The norm is to continue to hand us prescriptions for OAB, antibiotics or narcotics.

18. When you begin to improve discuss with your physician any changes in your medication regimen. Often the wonderful stable period of less pelvic pain goes off the tracks because the lining of the bladder always needs protection and genetically speaking, I know my bladder requires time to heal.

19. Do not shrug off increased symptoms.

20. BPS/IC does not go away. I think it is an allergic/inflammation response that delays the bladder lining cell replacement. All medicine offers is symptom control while we work on making our body environment as friendly as possible for healing.

Twenty people have written about their individual journeys and their discoveries to help you make sense of the chaotic condition of BPS/IC. Each person has taken the steps to recover from bladder caused urge, frequency, and pain to help you take greater control of your BPS/IC.

You are not alone.

Edward L. Davis, M.D.
Jo Davis, R.N, B.S.N., C.R.C.
Citrus Valley IC Support Group, Inc.

Acknowledgements

Joan King was the first to see that a collection of first-person accounts about BPS/IC could help others in search of answers. By writing about two of her five children who have IC, she added her parenting wisdom and how family life influences BPS/IC. Her steady patient advocacy for both the IC Clinic & Support Group has added quality of life issues as a major component to understanding the impact of pelvic pain.

Grace Perez took boxes of BPS/IC information and put them in order. She did this while going through chemo and radiation therapy. With a little help, she wrote about BPS/IC and cancer treatments. We hope we presented her personal story of dealing with what life hands you as clear as she would want it to be. We miss her.

Lisa Regan, C.R.C. said fourteen years ago that IC was not going to be the center of her life. For thirteen years, she has been at the center of Citrus Valley Medical Research, Inc. and the BPS/IC Clinic. Lisa has listened on the detailed research level of how men and women deal with BPS/IC; we have benefited from her knowledge.

Aaron Davis is one of our sons and a partner of Metabolic Markets, LLC (www.metabolicmarkets.com). He gathered the BPS/IC narratives and wondered why we were not moving forward with publishing. He took the information and started us down the road to deliver this information to you. Aaron was the editor we so needed.

Lynne Arciero is the managing director of the marketing firm Positraction, Inc. (www.positraciton.com). She provided the graphics resource that took the passion of the individual accounts and translated it into a cover that says so much about how we live our lives.

Linda Laubach, B.S.N., R.N., C.C.M. & Linda Bruner volunteered their time to provide copy editing direction and recommendations. We are grateful for their time and focus.

Thank you,

Edward Davis, M.D. – Jo Davis

Made in United States
Orlando, FL
10 March 2023

30900195R00130